The Diet Doctors

Inside and Out
The ULTIMATE 12-Week Diet Plan

Dr Samina Showghi, Pam Stepney
and Dr Ben King

with Dr Diane Storey

HarperCollins*Publishers*

'Dedicated to our loving families, both near and far'

HarperCollins*Publishers*
77–85 Fulham Palace Road
Hammersmith, London W6 8JB

The website address is: www.harpercollins.co.uk

First published by HarperCollins 2008

10 9 8 7 6 5 4 3 2 1

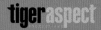

an I⅃∖G media company

© Tiger Aspect Productions Limited 2008

Dr Samina Showghi, Pam Stepney, Dr Ben King and Dr Diane Storey
have asserted their moral right to be identified as the authors of this work

Photograph p.iv © John Wright/Amarang.com
All other photographs © Mark Read

Stylist: Rachel Jukes
Food stylist: Fergal Connolly

A catalogue record of this book is
available from the British Library

ISBN-13 978-0-00-727057-6
ISBN-10 0-00-727057-7

Printed and bound in Great Britain by
Butler and Tanner, Somerset

Contents

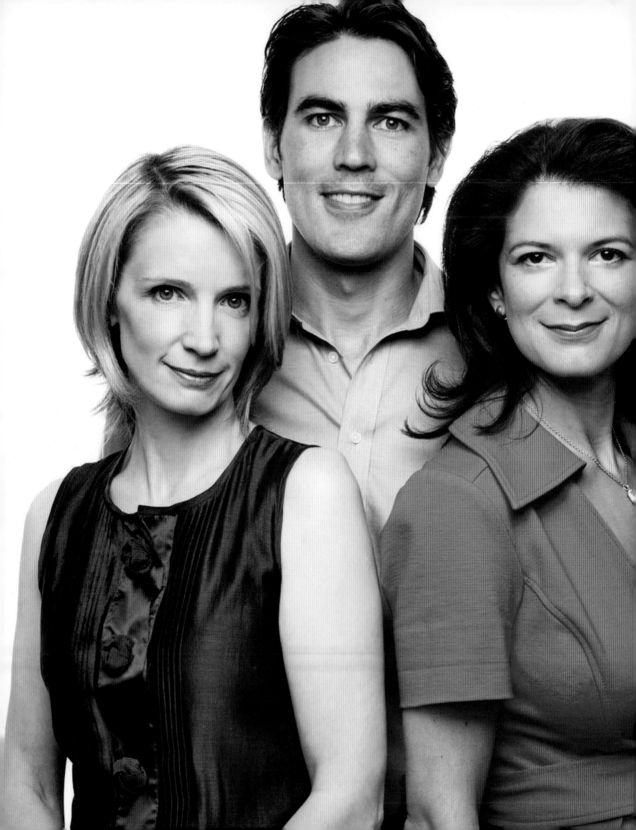

We can change your life

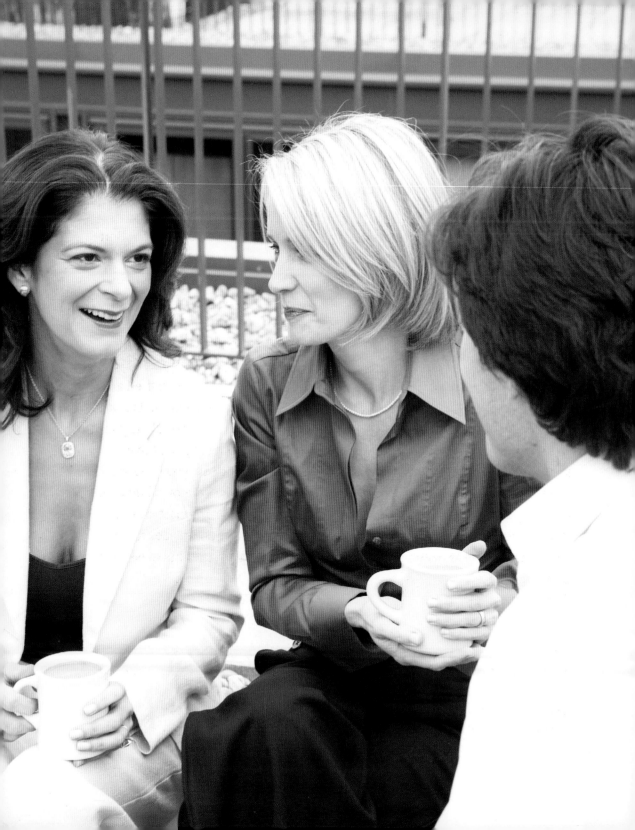

Are you fed up with dieting? Have you tried everything going – high protein, low carb, meal replacements, food combining? There are masses of diets to try but most are very restrictive. You can't follow them for life and so they won't work long term. Chances are you'll end up putting all the weight back on, and then some. But that won't stop you trying another diet and so the yo-yo diet cycle continues. It's a vicious circle, a fat trap that you need to escape now.

You do have a choice. You don't have to carry on living with the body you have now. You can change your lifestyle and lose weight in a healthy way. You can slim down, and stay that way forever. Every day, we help disillusioned dieters lose weight and turn their lives around. We see the results – they look better, feel great and shed health problems along with the excess weight. We help them, both inside and out.

We can help you and this book is your personal consultation. We will be with you, week by week, every step of the way. This book shows you how, in just 12 weeks, you can get your body back in shape and get back on track to a healthier future. BUT it's not a short term fix. We haven't designed it to be a rigid, strict plan that has to be endured. Food should taste great and exercise should be pleasurable. This is a plan you need to embrace – it should fit into your lifestyle. You can't abandon it when you've shifted a few stones – nor should you want to. It's a flexible plan, which will allow you treats but if you really want to look good inside and out, you have to take responsibility for your own body. Be balanced in your approach to exercise and eating and you will look and feel like a million dollars – but even more importantly, we believe, you'll be healthy inside too.

Dr Samina Showghi
GP, MBBS MRCGP DCH DRCOG

Pam Stepney
Nutritionist, B.Sc.

Dr Ben King
Chiropractor, B.Sc., M.Chiro

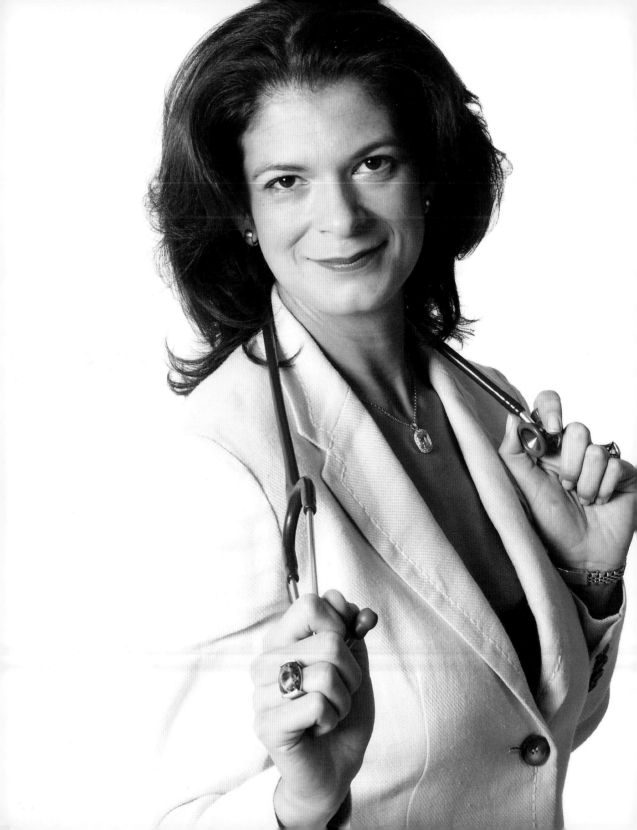

CHAPTER 1

The Doctors are ready for you now ...

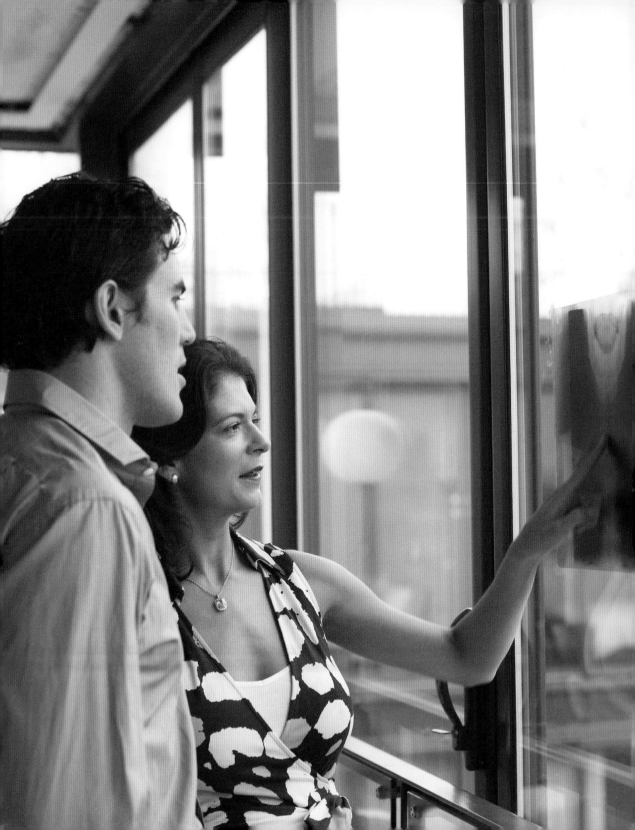

Checkup

Bodies need a bit of looking after, so they look good and perform well. Reading this book suggests that you are already aware that something's not quite right – perhaps you're rather out of shape and you're wondering what to do about it?

And of course, the way your body looks on the outside closely reflects how well things are going under the skin, on the inside. Get everything sorted on the inside, and problems on the outside often get solved without really trying. So even though your main aim may be to look good on the beach, to drop a dress size or to wow everybody at a wedding, the 12-week diet plan focuses on the inside.

Let's start with a checkup, beginning with your appearance. The outside gives important clues about what's going on inside, and we want you to be healthy. It's as much about feeling good as looking good. So have a look in the mirror and answer the questions over the page as honestly as you can.

Don't worry if there seems to be a lot of them. They're simple questions and it's important to get an overall view of your health and wellbeing. Just tick the yes/no boxes, and fill in any details.

'I'm constantly amazed at the body's capacity to heal itself.' DR SAMINA

Checklist for healthy appearance

	No	Yes	Details

SKIN

Do you often have sores or ulcers?

Do you suffer from greasy, spotty skin?

Does your skin bruise easily?

Does your skin often itch, or feel dry
and flaky?

HAIR

Have you got excessive hair loss, either
from all over your head or in patches?

Have you got excessive hair growth?
If so, where?

Has your hair changed in amount or
texture recently?

NAILS ON FINGERS AND TOES

Have your nails changed in appearance,
shape or texture?

Are your nails brittle or do they often
peel or break?

	No	Yes	Details

EYES

Do your eyes feel dry or itchy?

Do you experience difficulty seeing when it is dark or have night blindness?

Are there any raised yellow bumpy spots around your eyes, or a white ring round the coloured part of your eye?

MOUTH AND THROAT

Do your gums bleed when you clean your teeth?

Does your breath smell unpleasant?

Is there a scummy look to your tongue, or is your tongue red and cracked?

POSTURE, STANDING HOW YOU USUALLY STAND

When you look at yourself sideways in a full-length mirror, is the back of your head forward of your heels?

Again, looking at your side view, does your backside stick out?

Does your belly stick out?

Do your shoulders jut forwards?

Looking face on to the mirror, are your hips at different levels?

Does one leg look longer than the other?

The next thing is weighing and measuring. If you're serious about losing weight, we need to find out what the situation is now – and then just think how good it will be to see the improvement. So it's worth getting on the scales as things are going to get better.

Throughout the plan we're going to ask you to weigh yourself once a week, and once a week only. It doesn't really matter what time of day you weigh yourself, but you will weigh slightly less in the morning than you do in the evening. Choose a time when you will be able to weigh yourself regularly and consistently with (or without) clothes.

We also need to know your body measurements – and again, knowing what they are now means you'll have the satisfaction of seeing them get smaller as you follow our 12-week diet plan.

We'll be asking you to measure yourself every week too. Make sure when you measure that you are not holding your breath in or breathing out excessively, just breathe naturally. Measure where the tape is snug against your body – not pulled too tight. Measure your chest around the fullest part. Then measure your waist. The easiest way to make sure that you measure your waist in a consistent way is to put the tape measure round at the level of your belly button. Again, don't pull it tight, but measure where it is a snug fit. Then measure across the widest part of your hips and backside. If you want to, you can measure round your thighs, or any other parts of your body (upper arm? calf? neck?) that you are particularly concerned about.

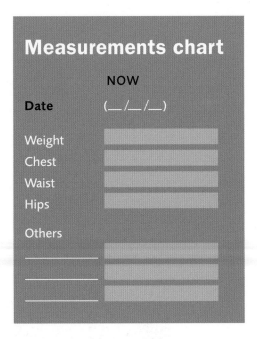

Measurements chart

	NOW
Date	(__ /__ /__)
Weight	
Chest	
Waist	
Hips	
Others	
_____	
_____	
_____	

Write down your weight, and the other measurements you've taken, in the table opposite. It doesn't matter if you prefer imperial measurements (stones, pounds, feet and inches) or metric (kilograms and centimetres), but just stick to one or the other.

All that remains now is to ask you about your personal history. It won't take long but gives a good clear picture as a starting point. As before, just tick the boxes, and fill in any relevant details.

Health history checklist

	No	Yes	Don't Know	Details

HEART AND CIRCULATION

▶ Do you have high blood pressure? ☐ ☐ ☐

▶ Do you have high cholesterol levels? ☐ ☐ ☐

▶ Have you ever had heart or circulation problems? ☐ ☐ ☐

DIGESTIVE SYSTEM

▶ Do you suffer from heartburn or indigestion? ☐ ☐ ☐

▶ Do you often have diarrhoea or constipation? ☐ ☐ ☐

▶ Is there ever blood in your stool? ☐ ☐ ☐

MUSCLES AND BONES

▶ Do you have muscle cramping or pain? ☐ ☐ ☐

▶ Do you have muscle wasting or weakness? ☐ ☐ ☐

▶ Do you have osteoporosis or bone fractures? ☐ ☐ ☐

▶ Do you have arthritis or joint problems? ☐ ☐ ☐

	No	Yes	Don't Know	Details

OTHERS

▶ Are you often tired or fatigued without reason?

▶ Do you suffer from headaches?

▶ Do you have weakness or tingling in your fingers or elsewhere?

▶ Is your libido low?

▶ Do you often feel depressed or irritable, or find it hard to concentrate?

▶ Has your weight changed markedly in recent years?

So we've now got a fairly full picture of your current appearance and health. So what does it all mean?

Don't worry if …

Look back at the answers you've filled in. If you could answer 'no' to all the questions on appearance and on your health history, then the signs are looking very good that you are pretty healthy – though of course, if there is anything about your health that you *are* worried about, you should see your GP.

What about your weight? Is it a healthy weight for your height? You probably instinctively know if it is the right weight for you. But we can also work out your body mass index (often shortened to BMI) to see if your weight is in the healthy range for your height. To work out your BMI, you need to measure your height. Then using the chart below, simply run a finger along the line corresponding to your height, and another finger along the line that corresponds to your weight. The point where the two lines cross is your BMI.

If it is in the green section of the graph (BMI of 18.5–25), then your weight is within the healthy range for your height.

Sometimes, the BMI chart can suggest that you are overweight when you are actually rather athletic and muscular – this applies particularly to athletic men. That's because muscle weighs more than fat. Dr Ben has a few words to say about this: 'I'm 90kg in weight and 189cm tall – in "old money", I'm around 14 stone 2 pounds, and just under 6 foot 3. On the chart, it means I'm in the overweight section, with a BMI just over 25. But I'm muscular from all the rugby playing I used to do in the past, and I'm still active every day through my work and exercise. If you've seen *The Diet Doctors: Inside and Out* programmes, or been to my clinic, you'll know I'm not overweight – I'm fit and healthy, as shown by my waist measurement of 34 inches.'

One way that we check if the BMI is giving a false assessment of being overweight is to look at the waist measurement. That's one of the reasons why we asked you to measure your waist. Like Dr Ben, you're unlikely to be overweight or obese if you are a man with a waist measurement of less than 37 inches or 94cm. If you are a woman, you are probably not overweight or obese if your waist measurement is less than 32 inches or 81cm.

So, if the checkup showed that you don't need to worry, what next? You could decide that you don't want to do anything differently, as your current lifestyle may not be causing you any harm. Or you might know, in your heart of hearts, that you could improve your diet and exercise routines. Our 12-week diet plan is all about becoming healthier. If you are already the right weight, you won't end up like a matchstick – you'll just have hair, eyes and skin that look even more glowing and healthy!

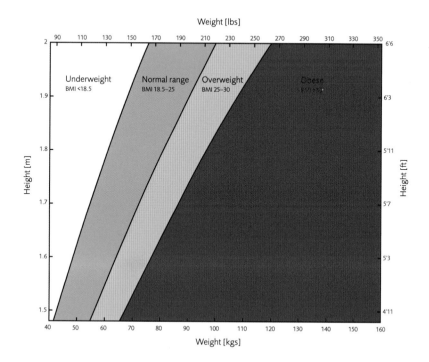

Worry if …

If your BMI is in the amber (overweight) or red (obese) areas of the chart, perhaps you should be concerned. Perhaps it's time for you to do something about losing weight. We'll help you. Our 12-week diet plan can get you started on losing weight, and is healthy enough to continue for life.

What about the rest of the checkup? Did you answer 'yes' to any of the healthy appearance questions? If so, it's likely that your body is trying to tell you that you are not looking after it properly. Your appearance is intimately linked with how you treat your body. Giving your body what it needs to function in a healthy way can work wonders for your overall appearance. Getting your posture right so that you stand tall gives your lungs a chance to work well and helps with those niggling aches and pains. Eating well nourishes your body, bringing energy and vitality. Follow our 12-week plan, and see for yourself how your appearance improves.

We know that extra weight causes a lot of heartache, and we don't just mean about going up a dress size or being too round to look good in a dinner jacket! We know that most strokes and heart attacks could be prevented with simple changes in the way people live their lives. We know that being obese increases the risk of getting some forms of cancer and shortens lives.

Getting your weight down to a healthy range by eating sensibly and well can help you live longer. And it's not just about living longer, but also about living better and feeling great. Just how much fun is it to be unable to move around, unable to do what you want, or to feel unable to go to a party because you're embarrassed about your weight?

You can enjoy life much more when you're healthy, fit and active. Look forward to having more energy, more opportunities, more life!

What do you want?

So what do you want to do? It helps to have a clear idea of what you want to achieve. But it's also important to be realistic about your goals. If what you want is a quick fix, think again. Surely, what you want is a real solution, to be slim and healthy? And yes, it is possible. A weight loss of 1–2lb a week (up to 1kg) is achievable in a healthy way. Over the next 12 weeks, you could lose between 1 and 2 stone in weight (around 10kg). Use the 'Goal' section in the chart below to record what you hope to achieve – and remember to add the date for when you want to reach the goal.

Having decided what you want, how are you going to get it? One thing is certain: if you don't change anything, you won't end up where you want to be. You may need to make significant changes to the way you eat. You may need to stop being a couch potato and get that body moving.

Give our suggestions a try during the next 12 weeks, and use the 'Help!' sections to give you the strength to keep going. Believe us, it does get easier! And once you achieve your goals, you will feel very encouraged to continue.

Measurements chart

	NOW	GOAL
Date	(__ /__ /__)	(__ /__ /__)
Weight		
Chest		
Waist		
Hips		
Others		
_____		
_____		
_____		

'No matter where you are now, it's never too late to be your ideal weight.' DR BEN

ULTIMATE 12-WEEK DIET PLAN

Our 12-week diet plan can get you started on losing weight. Our plan is also so healthy that you can follow it for life – no fads, no drastic measures, no impossible food bans. It's completely in line with accepted guidelines for healthy eating and exercising. You shouldn't be hungry, either – you're allowed a couple of snacks each day as well as three meals.

The 12-week diet plan includes a gradually increasing exercise programme, starting with improving the range of movement in all your joints, then moving on to exercises that improve heart and circulation, and finally increasing general strength. Don't be put off by the idea of exercising – if it's any comfort, none of us are gym bunnies, though we have all found ways of making exercise an enjoyable part of our lives. There's just no other way of keeping your body firing on all cylinders until you get that telegram on your 100th birthday!

The 12-week diet plan will improve your nutrition and flexibility, and can help resolve many health problems. But as you go through the plan, Dr Samina will mention things that could be of particular interest if you suffer from any specific problems with appearance or health, Pam will recommend specific foods to eat or avoid, and Dr Ben will give you exercises that can help you. But in case you can't wait, we've listed the pages that might be particularly relevant to you.

Our 12-week diet plan can get you started on losing weight. Our plan is also so healthy that you can follow it for life – no fads, no drastic measures, no impossible food bans.

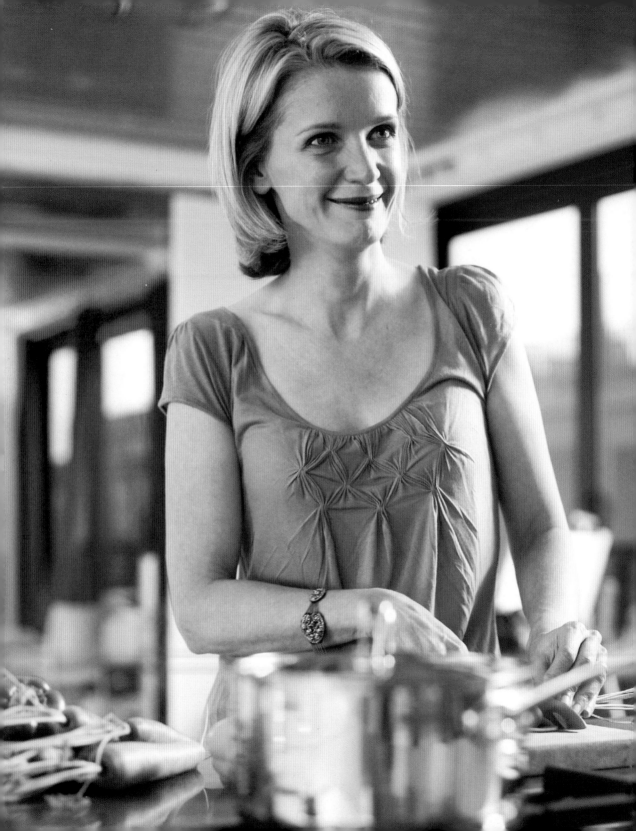

'Help!'

Let's face it, if you've ever tried to lose weight, you know it's not all plain sailing. There'll be days when you'll be tempted to give up and go back to your old ways. We said we're here to help you week by week and we are.

The chances are, you'll face problems and temptations that we've seen before. Each week, we'll help you with these common problems. But in case a problem strikes early, here's a list of where you can find our help.

So what are you waiting for? The 12-week diet plan is going to help you shape up. You'll be fitter and healthier and more able to live the life you want to lead.

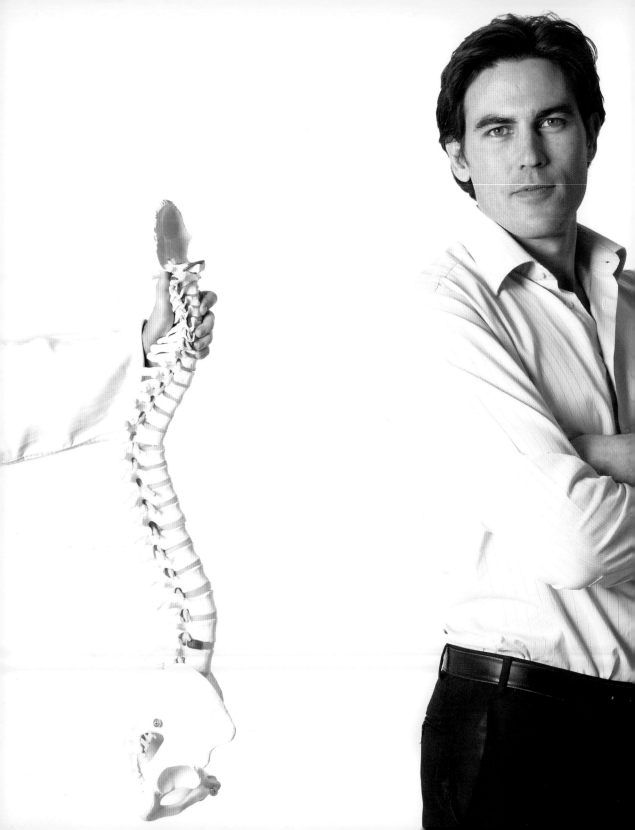

CHAPTER 2

First things first

Dear diary ...

The key to losing weight is changing the balance between how much you eat and how much energy your body uses up. All food contains energy (measured in calories) that is released when you digest it, and used up by your body as you move around. If you use up less energy than you eat, the extra is stored as fat. To get rid of the fat, you have to use up more energy than you eat, either by eating less or being more active, or ideally by doing both. Different foods contain different amounts of energy, so another way of losing weight is eating more food that's low in calories and less food that's high in calories. It is also important to space out your meals and not to eat all your calories for the day in one go.

Before you can decide what changes you need to make to be able to lose weight, you need to know what you are doing now. Do you *really* know what you are eating and drinking? As you may know from watching *The Diet Doctors: Inside and Out*, this is an important starting point for all the people we help, and it is important for you, too. Only when you see what you're doing now do you know what you want to change.

Just as we ask the people we help on the TV programme, we'd like you to keep a food diary for the next week. Get yourself a little notebook and record everything you eat and drink, and the time that you ate or drank it. Write down as much information as possible – it's not much help to write down bread, without saying how much, so write down if it was four slices thickly spread with butter and jam, or half a slice of granary bread with a scraping of peanut butter. Don't just write down 'cup of coffee'; give the complete picture and record any sugar or milk you add, as there's a big difference between a cup of black coffee and a creamy cappuccino. And don't forget to include drinks – alcoholic and non-alcoholic.

Remember to be honest. You are less likely to 'forget' that biscuit with your morning coffee if you keep the diary with you and write things down immediately. And yes, that means all those sneaky nibbles as you prepared the children's packed lunches, and the leftovers from their suppers! And don't forget the poppadoms that arrived on your table and just disappeared while you waited for your Indian meal to be served. What we are looking for is the complete picture – whatever it really is.

Record how you felt each time you ate or drank something, as well. Were you hungry when you ate the muffin at the coffee bar when you were out shopping with a friend, or did you just fancy it?

Were you plain hungry when you ate the bar of chocolate on your way home from work, or angry and frustrated after an irritating day in the office? Were you hungry an hour after your dinner when you started on the toast and jam, or just bored? Whatever your mood, jot it down.

We'll leave you to get on with the diary for the next week, and then we'll have a look at what it says about your current eating habits. We'll be asking you to keep a food diary throughout the 12-week plan to help you stay on track.

In the meantime, something that might help you as you fill in the diary is to think about portion sizes.

'Identifying any "trigger" foods is an important step in making changes – so keep a food diary.' PAM

Portion distortion

As well as *what* you're eating, we've asked you to record in your food diary how *much* food you're eating. We want you to notice the size of the portions you are having. That's because of a common problem – portion distortion. In the last 30 years, average portion sizes have grown by about a third, so that people often underestimate the number of calories they are eating. No wonder so many people have put on weight!

To make sure that what *you* call a portion is the same as what *we* call a portion, let's get rid of portion distortion. Here is what Pam has to say about portions:

'When is a portion not a portion? When it's a heap or a mountain! But joking aside, it's quite easy to know that a mountain of food is really much bigger than the portion you need, but it's less obvious when it genuinely seems like a small amount. It makes sense to start thinking about what kind of food you are eating, and how much you are having. So use my guidelines on portions as you keep your food diary, and later on when you start on the 12-week diet plan. Don't worry though, I don't mean you'll need to do this every day and for every meal – just until you can gauge by eye the right amount for a portion.

'Later, I'll give you guidance on how much of each type of food to eat to help you lose weight and feel great. Try not to stock up the fridge and cupboards again until you've completed the diary and considered what it all means.'

A portion of fruit or vegetables is the amount that's the size of your fist. That means one portion is a big apple, a fist-sized bunch of grapes, or a couple of plums. If you've got a cup or bowl about the size of your fist, try using this to measure a portion. Fill it up with lettuce leaves, for example, and then tip it out to see what the portion looks like.

A portion of rice, pasta or potato is the size of a small grapefruit. We're not talking a steaming plateful of spaghetti as one portion! Look in your cupboards and find a bowl, about the size of a small grapefruit and use this as a measure. Once it's cooked, a portion of rice, pasta or potato weighs about 150g.

A portion of bread is one slice.

A portion of meat or fish is the size of a pack of playing cards. That means a small chicken breast is one portion. A chunky steak that covers most of the plate will be two or even three portions.

One sausage or two rashers of bacon is one portion.

A portion of nuts is about five brazils, or about 10 almonds, pecans or walnuts or a handful of peanuts.

A portion of milk is half a pint, a portion of yoghurt is one small pot and a single egg counts as a portion.

A portion of cheese is the size of a matchbox (about 30g – 125 calories). Again, try putting this amount on a plate and see what it looks like. A typical bought cheese sandwich contains about one and a half portions of cheese – about 45g. Remember that although cheese is a nutritious food, it also usually contains a lot of fat, making it high in calories.

A small packet of crisps (25–30g) counts as a portion, and so does a small slice of cake (25g), a 25g handful of sweets or a few squares of chocolate. Two biscuits count as a portion.

Limber up

There's something else you can do this week, while you're completing your food diary – you can see how well your body moves. As you lose weight, you will want to *feel* good in your body, as well as *look* good. As with looking at your food intake, it's useful to know the starting point. You can check out your flexibility using some simple exercises. They are designed to assess your body in a very gentle way, so should not cause any difficulties, but if you have any concerns, ask your doctor first.

Wearing comfortable clothing and with bare feet, warm up a little first with some gentle body movements like swinging your arms and walking on the spot. Then try out the following flexibility exercises. Don't bounce to try and reach further as you might hurt yourself. Just tick the box showing where you can comfortably reach with each exercise. It might be easier if you have someone to help you check how far you can reach and to tick the boxes for you, but if that's not possible, try the exercises in front of a mirror so you can assess yourself.

'We are not immortal, we have an expiry date – so stop wasting your life, you don't have time! Get fit and healthy, and start enjoying life.' DR BEN

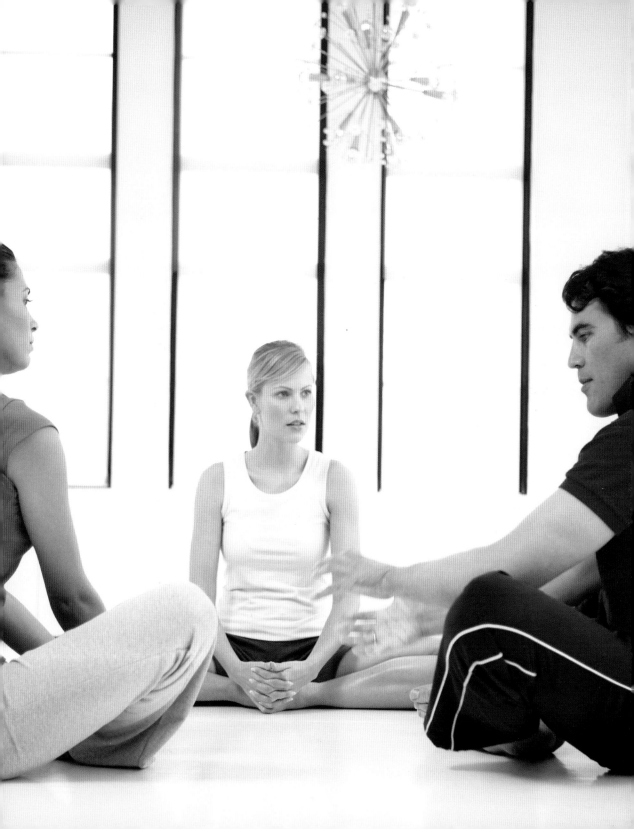

Flexibility test

	1 POINT	2 POINTS	3 POINTS
1 Standing up straight with your feet flat on the floor and straight legs, bend sideways letting your hand glide down your leg without leaning forwards or backwards. How far can you reach? Try both sides. If there is a difference, score for the side that has the least reach.	Thigh ☐	Knee ☐	Lower leg ☐
2 Standing up straight with your feet flat on the floor, keep your arms straight out at shoulder level and try to cross them over in front of you. Where do your arms cross? Try right arm over left, and left arm over right, and if there is a difference between sides, score for the side that crosses lowest down your arm.	Wrist ☐	Elbow ☐	Upper arm ☐
3 Standing up, put one arm up above your head and the other hanging down by your side. Bend both arms towards your back and try to reach your hands together behind you. Do your fingers reach? If not, how far apart are they? Switch sides, so that the other arm is high. If there is a difference, score for the side that has the biggest gap between hands.	Fingers more than 6 inches (15cm) apart ☐	Fingers less than 6 inches (15cm) apart ☐	Fingers meet ☐
4 Sit down on a hard, upright chair, with your hands on your knees. Keeping your backside pushed into the back of the chair, try bending your trunk forwards, letting your hands move towards your feet. How far do your hands go?	Fingers do not reach the floor ☐	Fingers reach the floor ☐	Hands flat on the floor ☐

	1 POINT	2 POINTS	3 POINTS
5 Sit down on the floor with the soles of your feet together and your knees open. Gently press your knees open and down towards the floor. How far do they comfortably reach?	More than 6 inches (15cm) ☐	About 6 inches from the floor ☐	Less than 6 inches from the floor ☐
6 Still on the floor, stretch out your legs in front of you and, with straight knees, reach towards your toes. How far can you go?	More than 6 inches from toes ☐	Less than 6 inches from toes ☐	Touch toes ☐
7 Lie down flat on the floor on your back. Keeping one leg straight, bend the other knee towards your chest. How close can it get? Now straighten that leg and try bending the other knee. If there is a difference between sides, score for the leg that stays the furthest from your chest.	Knee more than 6 inches from chest ☐	Knee less than 6 inches from chest ☐	Knee touches the chest ☐
8 Still on your back, bend both knees, keeping your feet flat on the floor and stretch out your arms on the floor at either side. Lower your knees towards the floor on one side of your body, without your shoulders coming off the floor. How close do your knees get? Try the other side. If there is a difference, score for the side that stays the furthest from the floor.	Knee more than 6 inches from floor ☐	Knee less than 6 inches from floor ☐	Knee reach the floor ☐

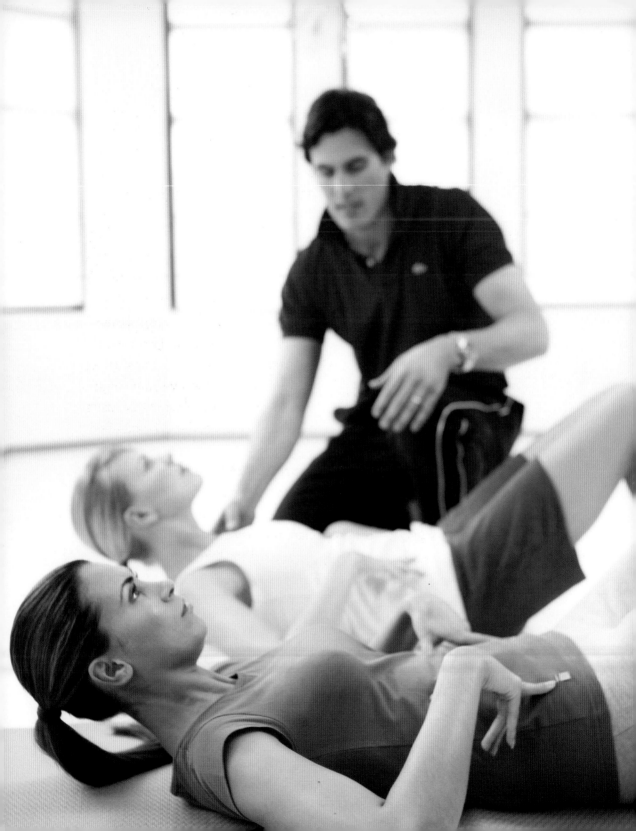

Add up your total score and jot it down below, with the date. How did you get on?

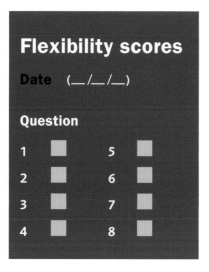

Flexibility scores

Date (__/__/__)

Question

1	☐	5	☐
2	☐	6	☐
3	☐	7	☐
4	☐	8	☐

Score 8–13? You are not very flexible at the moment. You might benefit from seeing a chiropractor to check out any body misalignments, particularly if the health check in the last chapter showed that your posture could be improved.

Score 14–18? You are reasonably flexible, but there may be room for improvement. Did you score highly on some exercises and low on others, or were you in the middle for most of the exercises? It could be that you need all-round help to improve your range of movements, or you might have parts of the body that need special attention.

Score 19–24? You are already very flexible. You should have no problems with the first stage of the 12-week diet plan, and may be able to bring forward the second and third sections of the exercise plan.

At the end of each four-week period, you will be able to check your flexibility again and feel great about the progress you've made.

What's the score?

Once you've completed your food diary for a week, it's time to have a look at what it all means. You may have seen what we do with the information from the food diaries completed by the people we help on *The Diet Doctors: Inside and Out*. We collect together all the food and drink recorded in the completed food diary to show the contributors what they are eating.

You could get a similar effect by looking at what you buy in your weekly shopping. Of course, the main problem with doing this at home is that you may not shop weekly, so you might not have the chance to see all that you eat in one go. You may often have takeaways or eat out at cafés, restaurants, pubs or the work canteen, or buy snacks when you are out and about, eating them immediately. This is where the diary comes in handy.

Look at your completed diary and divide up the food you have eaten into five groups.

GROUP 1

Fruit and vegetables (including fresh and frozen, dried fruit, fruit juice, beans and pulses)

GROUP 2

Bread, cereals, potatoes, rice and pasta

GROUP 3

Meat, fish and other protein-rich foods (including eggs and nuts)

GROUP 4

Milk and dairy foods (including cheese and yoghurt, but not including butter, eggs or cream)

GROUP 5

High-fat foods (including butter, cream, margarine, mayonnaise, chocolate, crisps, rich sauces, gravy) and high-sugar foods (including soft drinks, sweets, jam, sugar, cakes, biscuits, pastries, ice cream).

Count up how many portions of each of the five groups you ate each day. Now use the information from your diary to assess your healthy eating score.

Healthy eating questionnaire

	YES	USUALLY	NO
GROUP 1 (fruit and vegetables)			
Did you eat 5 portions of group 1 food on most days?	A	B	C
Did you eat less than 3 portions of group 1 food on most days?	C	B	A
Do fruit and vegetables make up half of all your daily food and drink?	A	B	C
Do fruit and vegetables make up less than a third of all your daily food and drink?	C	B	A
GROUP 2 (bread, cereals, potatoes, rice and pasta)			
Did you eat more than five portions of group 2 foods?	C	B	A
Did bread, cereals, potatoes, rice or pasta make up less than a third of all your daily food?	A	B	C
Were less than half of your portions of bread, rice and pasta wholegrain, granary, brown or wholewheat?	C	B	A
GROUP 3 (meat, fish, nuts, eggs)			
Did you eat more than five portions of group 3 foods on most days ?	A	B	C
Did burgers, bacon, sausage, ham or ready meals make up more than a third of your portions of meat and fish?	C	B	A
Did you eat more than two portions of fish during the week?	A	B	C
Did you eat more than two portions of nuts during the week?	A	B	C
GROUP 4 (milk and dairy)			
Did you eat more than four portions of group 4 foods on most days?	C	B	A
Did you usually use skimmed or semi-skimmed milk?	A	B	C
GROUP 5 (high fat, high sugar)			
Did you eat more than two portions of group 5 foods and drinks on most days?	C	B	A

Count up how many of each letter you circled. How did you get on?

Mostly As You're already eating well, though you can still improve. You may be eating all of the right things, in the right proportions, but if you want to lose weight you need to eat smaller portions and exercise more.

Mostly Bs You're eating reasonably well, but there may be room for improvement. Did you get more As and Bs in some areas and Cs in others, or were you in the middle for most of the assessments? There may be particular areas that need attention. Following the 12-week diet plan should help you circle more As. Your body should get slimmer, your health should improve and you should feel great.

Mostly Cs Your diet is not very healthy at the moment. You really need to get on our 12-week diet plan to start getting into shape and turning around your health.

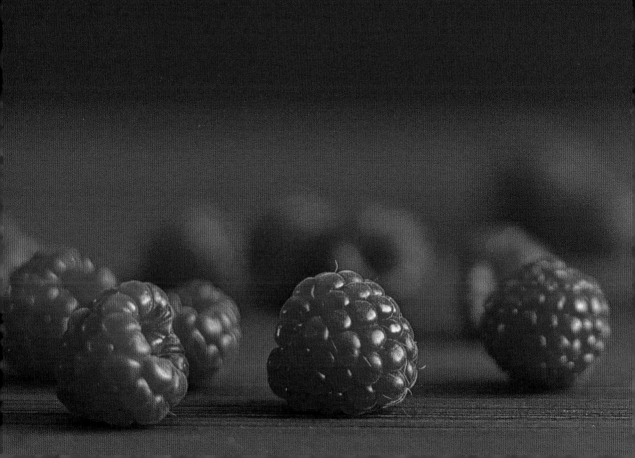

At the end of the 12-week period, you will be able to check your healthy eating habits again and feel great about the progress you've made.

'I tend to see three types of overweight people. Firstly, there's the group who just eat a little bit too much each day. Slowly their weight creeps up, without them really noticing, and then a year later they've gone up by a stone or more. These people need to take care with portion sizes, and also think about any habits they've got into that are adding too many calories – like a cake every day with their morning coffee, or takeaway fish and chips every week. Then there are the habitual dieters – people who regularly miss breakfast and lunch to try and cut down, but then overeat in the evening, so they should try to eat regularly. Lastly, I see binge-type eaters who focus on one food and can't stop eating it once they start. They need to avoid the trigger foods altogether and develop strategies for tackling the binges.' **PAM**

Eating well

If you eat the right quantity of food for the exercise you take, and you eat the right proportions of each group of food, you will be doing the best you can for your health and wellbeing. So what should you be aiming for?

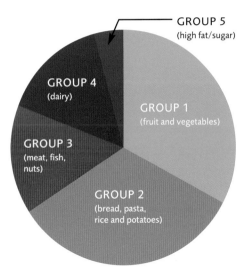

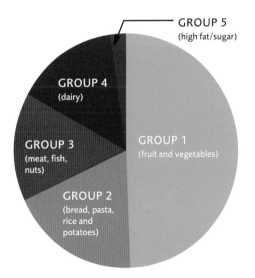

portions each day. Another third of your food should come from group 2 foods (bread, pasta, rice or potatoes). Of the remaining food, it should be made up of group 3 foods (protein-rich foods like meat, fish and nuts), and group 4 foods (milk and dairy), with only a very small amount of group 5 foods each day.

The plate above shows the right proportions of food for someone who is already a healthy weight.

It shows that about a third of your daily food should come from group 1 foods (fruit and vegetables), with at least five

For someone who is overweight, the proportion of group 2 foods should be reduced, and replaced with more fruit and vegetables as shown in the chart above. This means that about half of

your daily food should come from fruit and vegetables, and less than a third from bread, pasta, rice or potatoes.

Your food diary and healthy eating score will give you a good indication of whether or not you're eating well. If not, you can see where the problem lies. We usually find that people eat far too many group 5 foods (high-calorie fatty and sugary foods like crisps, biscuits, cakes, ice cream, chocolate, sugar included in tea and coffee, and soft drinks), and not enough group 1 foods (fruit and vegetables).

There's also often a problem with the type of foods eaten within each group. Meat products that are high in fat, like ready meals and takeaways, mean these portions are packing far more calories than they should. They also contain saturated fats which have been linked to heart disease (see page 105). And eating only meat proteins means that you may be missing out on the other useful nutrients in other sources of protein (like fish and nuts). These protein sources contain unsaturated fats that are helpful for your heart, with

the essential omega unsaturated fats being particularly beneficial.

It's similar for dairy products. Pint for pint, skimmed or semi-skimmed milk contains half the calories of full fat, whilst still offering the goodness. And there's a world of difference between full-fat cream cheese and low-fat cottage cheese, without a great deal of difference in their flavour.

So what should you do about it? The 12-week diet plan is based on healthy eating so that you gradually shift your food to match the ideal. You will be encouraged to eat more fruit and vegetables, and maximize the goodness you get from the protein and dairy foods you eat. Although we don't ban anything, we want you to cut back on the high-fat and high-sugar foods you eat so these foods make a very minor contribution to what you are eating. We also want you to drop white, refined and processed group 2 foods, like white sliced bread and white rice, and switch to wholegrain or granary bread, wholewheat pasta and brown rice for maximum nutrients.

What's in the fridge?

OK, so you know what you need to do. What about taking the first step towards becoming slim for life? You might find this rather surprising, but we want you to take a trip to the kitchen. Go and have a look in the fridge and all the food cupboards.

What do you see? Do you see packs of ready meals waiting to be heated up in the microwave? Sausages, burgers and ham? A freezer full of pizzas topped with pepperoni and ham? White sliced bread? Packets of crisps, biscuits and cakes? If this is what you see, you'll find it hard to score well on the healthy eating assessment, but don't worry – we'll help your fridge get a makeover as well as you!

We're not going to ask you to throw away food that you've already bought – though if you don't fancy eating it any more, we'd be quite happy for you to get rid of it. The most important thing is not to buy more of the foods that make it difficult for you to lose weight and are not helping you become healthier.

By the end of the 12-week diet plan, when you look in your fridge you'll see food that will help you and your family eat well, so that you can become slim and healthy. There will be lean meat and fish waiting to be turned into healthy and fresh home-cooked meals. You'll see a vegetable drawer brimming with a wide range of colourful fresh produce, and a rainbow of fruit waiting to be eaten. Your fridge will contain skimmed or semi-skimmed milk, low-fat cheese, eggs and natural yoghurt. When you look in your bread bin, you'll find granary or wholegrain bread. In the food cupboard, there'll be tins of tuna and sardines ready to become quick suppers or tasty salads, and packets of nuts, seeds and dried fruits as handy snacks.

Supermarket sweep

Next time you shop, take a fresh approach to the supermarket aisles.

Stock up on fruit and vegetables and skip the aisles that will tempt you away from the plan.

- **Choose your fruit and veg first.** To begin with, select familiar ones like apples, pears and oranges or cabbage, broccoli and beans. You don't have to launch straight into aubergines or pak choi!

- **Veg on the go.** Think as well about vegetables that can make convenient snacks eaten raw –carrot and celery sticks, cherry tomatoes, cauliflower florets.

- **Think frozen.** Frozen vegetables are usually as nutritious as fresh ones. Peas and sweetcorn are great freezer staples and easy to slip into a meal if you're caught short.

- **Choose wholegrain or granary bread** instead of white sliced.

- **Buy brown rice and wholewheat pasta** to try out.

- **Buy skimmed or semi-skimmed milk.** Young children should stick to whole fat milk unless they are overweight.

- **Skip the aisles selling biscuits, chocolates, crisps and fizzy drinks.** If you don't go down them you'll be less tempted to slip them into your trolley.

- **Fish is the original fast food** – it doesn't only have to come from the chippie! Get some fresh fish or tins of tuna and salmon.

- **Don't buy any more ready-prepared meals.** There are many other ways of eating quickly when you get home from work without skimping on food quality.

- **Buy lean meat** (such as steak, skinless chicken breasts and lean mince to make into low-fat burgers) rather than sausages, bacon or ready-made burgers.

Getting in on the action

So you're ready now to get started on the first stage of the eating plan. You've stocked up on fruit, vegetables and healthy foods. What about getting ready for exercise? This is going to be a very short section – because you don't need to belong to a gym. You don't need a tracksuit or joggers. You don't even need a pair of trainers.

The only thing you may want to invest in is a pedometer. A simple and inexpensive one is fine – don't think you need to splash out on a fancy one! The most important thing is for you to start recognizing that moving your body is important if you want to control your weight and improve your health. Exercising while you are losing weight is also important as it makes sure that it's fat you lose, not muscle.

'Help! I hate the gym'

Don't worry, we don't like going to the gym either. Even Dr Ben, who loves fencing, boxing, rugby, running, swimming, Pilates, walking, salsa ... you name it, even he doesn't like going to the gym and you can't say he's not fit! The simple answer is that if you're embarrassed about going to the gym or don't know what to do there, it doesn't matter. You don't have to go to a gym to lose weight.

To begin with on the 12-week diet plan, we want you to get used to moving your body, to increase the range of movement in all your joints. You can do these movements in the privacy of your bedroom, with no need for anyone to see you, no need for special clothes and no risk of feeling self-conscious.

Only from Week 5 do we ask that you start exercising that rather important muscle – your heart. This will help it get stronger and better at pumping blood round your body, help nutrients flow round your body better, and help you lose weight by burning up energy. But it's your choice what kind of exercise you do. It might be something as simple as walking for half an hour every other day. It might be a trip to the park with the kids a couple of times a week for an energetic game of Frisbee or to kick a ball around. It might be joining a dancing class. There are plenty of enjoyable ways to exercise your heart and lungs.

We want you to enjoy whatever exercise you choose to do, so stop worrying, and get started on the first stage of the 12-week diet plan!

'The gym is a wonderful tool, with set classes and trainers to ask for advice. Some people find the gym a convenient and stress-free place to train but it's not your only option!' DR BEN

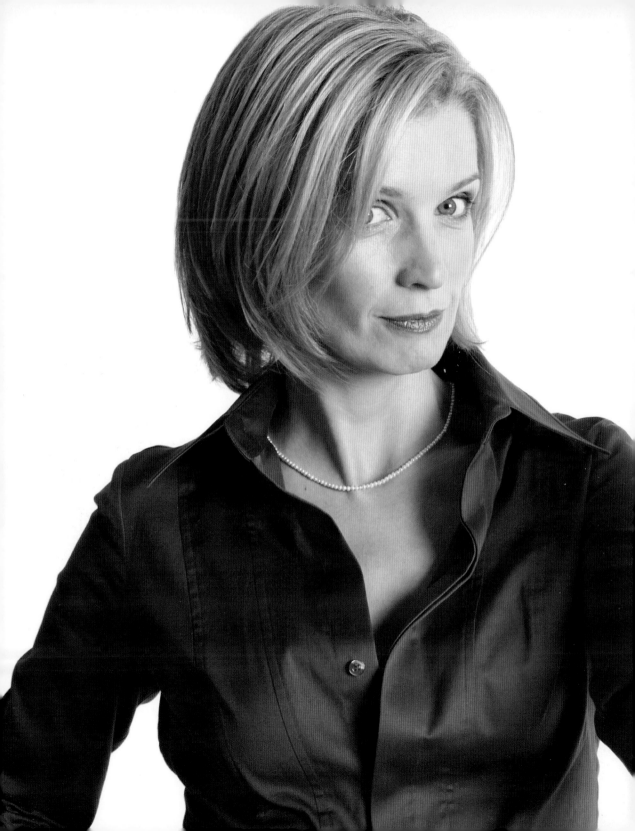

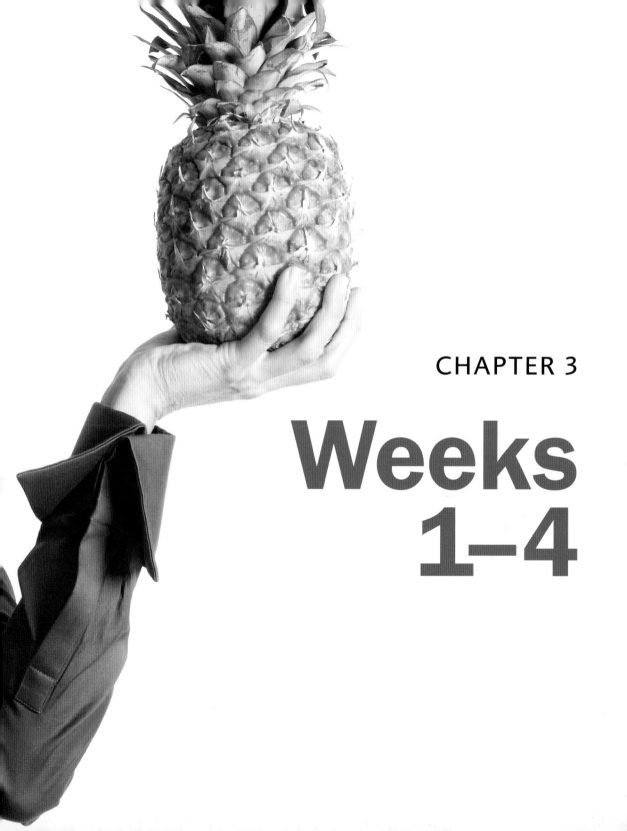

CHAPTER 3

Weeks 1-4

What's going to happen this month?

You're now ready to start on the 12-week diet plan. We're not going to give you a rigid day-by-day programme of exactly what to eat and when to exercise. That's because it wouldn't suit everyone and it would be impossible to stick to. Instead, we'll give you general rules that you can interpret in the way that suits your life. Follow these and you should lose 4–8lbs in weight during this first month.

So what exactly do we want you to do? Well, first of all you need to start making simple changes to your normal eating habits so your meals become healthier. We'll be giving you lots of ideas and recipes to choose from.

We want you to eat three meals and two healthy snacks every day and to include a little protein with each one. You also need to build up to eating five portions of fruit and veg each day and to limit yourself to no more than one portion of high-fat, high-sugar food a day – this means no more than a couple of squares of high quality chocolate, OR a small packet of crisps, OR a sliver of cake.

You also need to keep a close eye on your portion sizes – stick to Pam's guidelines on pages 26–27. Keep a food diary to help you, noting how you feel when you eat as well. This will help identify any unhealthy eating traps.

In terms of what you drink, make water a priority. This means whenever you feel thirsty, drink a glass of water instead of any other beverage. As for alcohol, take a break from it. If you must have a drink when socializing, limit yourself to no more than one small alcoholic drink a day (such as a small 125ml glass of wine or a small bottle of beer).

We also want to you get into the habit of moving more and to build up to walking 10,000 steps a day. Use a pedometer to help you.

Finally, make a weekly appointment to weigh and measure yourself and record the information in your notebook or in the space provided. Don't weigh yourself more often as it will distract you.

The rules for weeks 1–4

1. Eat three meals and two healthy snacks every day. Have a little protein at every meal and snack

2. Eat more fruit and vegetables, building up to five portions a day

3. Eat no more than one portion of high fat, high sugar food a day

4. Get rid of portion distortion

5. Start drinking water

6. Take a break from alcohol

7. Follow the Daily Stretching Routine on pages 60–61 every day

8. Aim to walk 10,000 steps a day

9. Weigh and measure yourself at the start of each week

10. Keep a food and mood diary

Week 1 2 3 4

Start the week

Use the space below to record your target weight, so you can see what you are aiming for. Then write down your current weight and body measurements.

Measurements chart

	NOW	GOAL
Date	(__ /__ /__)	(__ /__ /__)
Weight		
Chest		
Waist		
Hips		
Others		
_____		
_____		
_____		

This is going to be the first of your weekly appointments with yourself to weigh and measure your progress. It doesn't matter if you weigh or measure yourself with your clothes on or off or at the start or end of the day. Just make sure that, week by week, you weigh yourself at the same time and in the same way.

Avoid the temptation of weighing yourself any more frequently as your weight will fluctuate on a daily basis. What we are looking for is a bigger picture of your progress and once a week will provide just that.

The other thing we'd like you to do is take a photo of how you look now so you can compare it with how you look at the end of the plan.

What's on the menu?

We've based the eating plan during the next four weeks on your usual diet. Of course, if you make no changes, you won't lose any weight. You've got to reduce the amount of calories that you eat, so that you start using up some of the food energy stored as fat. The trick is to start with small changes that you can manage comfortably. Even small changes can make a significant difference to your usual calorie count. If you are ready to move on to the next stage before the four weeks are up, that's fine – the plan is very flexible and is designed for you to adapt to suit your life.

We want you to start by eating regularly. Getting into good eating habits can really help you lose weight. If you regularly starve yourself by hardly eating in the early part of the day but then feel so hungry that you gorge in the evening, you're putting your body under horrible strain. It has to keep adjusting to feast and famine. This kind of eating pattern can also contribute to digestive problems such as diarrhoea, constipation and bloating. So we want you to eat three meals a day (breakfast, lunch and dinner no later than 3 hours before you go to bed). And to make sure you don't get too hungry, we want you to eat two small healthy snacks (mid-morning and mid-afternoon) – we don't mean crisps or chocolate! So it's out with the crisps and cake ... and in with the fruit and nuts.

Easy wins

GET RID OF THESE	CHOOSE THESE INSTEAD
Full-fat milk	Skimmed or semi-skimmed milk
Sugar in tea or coffee	No sugar
White bread	Wholegrain or granary bread
Fizzy drinks and other soft drinks	Water

Breakfast

So what should you have for breakfast? This is probably the most important meal of the day. If you don't normally eat breakfast before you leave the house, get up a bit earlier to give yourself sufficient time, or eat less in the evening so that you are hungry and want to eat in the morning. If you can't face eating, at least have a protein shake or smoothie – see the recipes in the last chapter. If you do normally eat breakfast, see if you can make some small changes to make it a healthier meal.

CHANGE FROM THIS BREAKFAST...	TO THIS BREAKFAST...
No breakfast	Some breakfast! Any breakfast from this list or a protein shake or smoothie
Two slices of white bread toast, spread with butter, jam or marmalade	Two slices of wholegrain or granary toast, spread with peanut butter or cottage cheese
Bowl of cereal (such as cornflakes or Weetabix) topped with sugar, served with full fat milk	Weigh out 30g of your usual cereal and eat it with some fresh fruit (such as sliced banana) in place of sugar and with skimmed or semi-skimmed milk
Bowl of sugary cereal (such as ricicles, frosties, frosted shreddies) served with full fat milk	Change to a less sugary cereal, and have 30g of it with fruit, and skimmed or semi-skimmed milk
Fried egg with two slices of fried bread white bread, sausage and bacon	Scrambled, boiled or poached egg with two slices of wholegrain or granary toast, grilled mushrooms and tomatoes

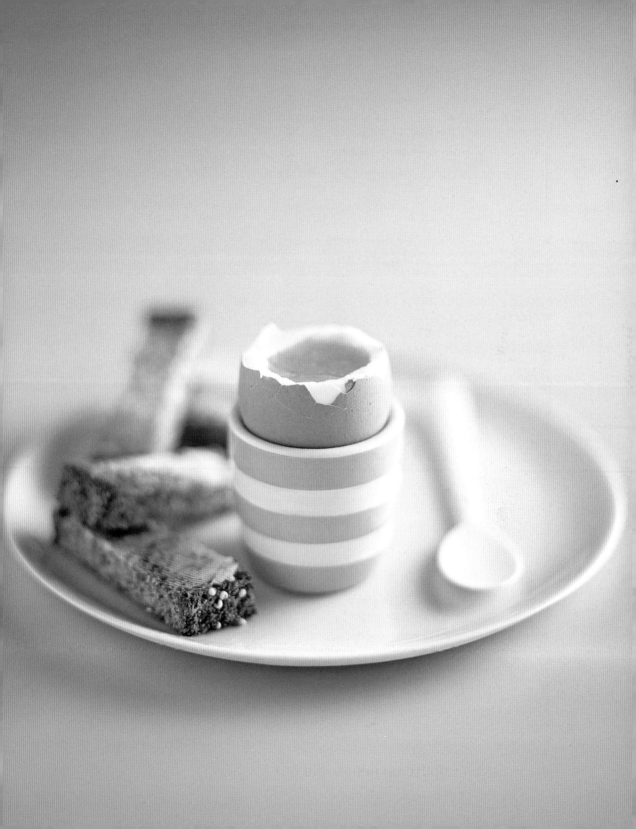

Lunch

Don't skip lunch, no matter how busy you are. As with your breakfast, we want you to make small changes to your usual lunch to cut down on the number of calories you have and to increase the nutritional value of your food.

CHANGE FROM THIS LUNCH...	TO THIS LUNCH...
Ham and pickle sandwich on white bread with crisps and a coke	Smoked salmon sandwich on wholemeal bread with cherry tomatoes and water
Large sausage roll, chocolate bar and mug of sweet milky coffee	Egg salad sandwich on granary bread with mug of herbal tea and handful of raisins
Tomato soup with croutons, a white roll and butter, followed by a doughnut	Tomato soup without the croutons, with a wholemeal roll and no butter, followed by fresh fruit salad
Large baked potato with butter, topped with tuna mayonnaise, followed by a muffin	Leafy green salad with tuna, cucumber, tomato and spring onions, followed by a natural yoghurt
Spaghetti bolognaise served with garlic bread and hot chocolate	Bolognaise sauce with half the usual amount of spaghetti, served with salad and fruit smoothie

Snacks

Your two small snacks are just as important as your three meals a day. This is because they will help control your hunger and at meal times you will feel satisfied eating a smaller portion. Don't be tempted to skip them in a bid to lose weight more quickly. So what sort of snacks do we mean? Sorry, not chocolate or crisps! We mean small bites that pack a nutritious punch.

GET RID OF THESE	CHOOSE THESE INSTEAD
Packet of crisps or savoury snacks	A pre-packed low-fat cheese (such as mini-Babybel Light or Laughing Cow light) and an apple
Chocolate bar	Small pot of natural yoghurt with some fruit added (such as a handful of strawberries, chopped pear)
Piece of cake or a few biscuits	2 oat cakes or crispbreads thinly spread with peanut butter
Bag of sweets	Banana and eight nuts
Hot chocolate and a muffin	Fruit smoothie and a few almonds

'Take a little self-seal plastic bag or box with you, containing your snacks. Don't get caught short, as that's when it's all too easy to go to the chocolate machine!' PAM

Dinner

When it comes to dinner, this month we just want you to adapt your usual meals so that you eat less of the rice, pasta or potato, and eat more vegetables. We want you to move away from ready meals and frozen convenience foods that are high in calories and low in nutrients, and towards healthy choices that help you eat well.

You should be able to adapt other meals that you normally cook. If you're having a roast dinner, just make sure that half your plate is filled with the vegetables, and have only one or two small roasties and a slice of meat less than you usually take. If you're having steak and chips, have only half your normal-sized piece of meat and just a few chips, and increase the amount of vegetables or salad so they take up half the space on the plate.

Cut out all the sugary food you may have as dessert after your dinner, or as snacks in the evening. Have fruit instead. If you are absolutely desperate for something sweet, a square or two of dark (70 per cent cocoa) chocolate should do the trick – not a big bar of milk or white chocolate.

CHANGE FROM THIS DINNER...	TO THIS DINNER...
8-inch pepperoni pizza with chips, followed by ice cream	Quarter of an 8-inch pizza with pepperoni removed and replaced with sliced tomato, chopped red pepper and tinned tuna, served with green leafy salad, followed by frozen yoghurt and chopped fruit, or try a healthy easy pizza (see recipe on page 192)
Six chicken nuggets with garlic bread, followed by chocolate cake	Chicken burger (see recipe on page 180) with green salad and sliced tomatoes, followed by fruit salad (see recipe on page 203)
Chicken curry ready meal with rice and naan bread, followed by cheese cake	Traditional balti chicken (see recipe on page 181) with 150g cooked rice, followed by natural yoghurt with fruit
Takeaway double cheese burger with mayonnaise in a white bun	Healthy burger with tomatoes and lettuce in a wholewheat bun (see recipe on page 191)
Frozen ready-prepared meatballs with chips	Meatballs in tomato sauce (see recipe on page 186)
Chip shop fish in batter with a large portion of chips	Pam's 'healthy' fish and chips (see recipe on page 170)
Shepherd's pie with potato topping	Shepherd's pie made with Pam's basic mince with hidden vegetables (see recipe on page 187)

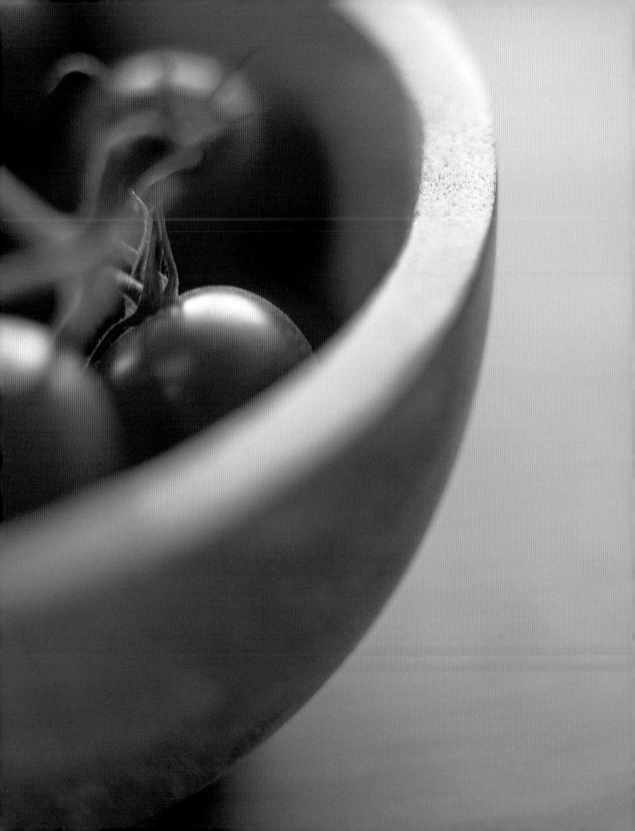

'Help! It'll all cost too much'

Don't worry, we won't blow your budget! If you're concerned about healthy food making an unhealthy dent in your purse or wallet, think about how much you're saving by no longer buying cakes, biscuits, crisps, chocolates, ready meals and takeaways – you'll find your money goes much further when you spend it on fruit, vegetables and ingredients for home cooking.

Remember that we're suggesting switching to things that are healthy versions of the same basic food, so cost around the same – skimmed or semi-skimmed milk instead of full-fat, wholegrain or granary bread instead of white sliced. And switching to tap water instead of drinking soft drinks can save you more than enough for extra fruit or veg, or steak instead of sausages!

Remember that we're also asking you to reduce how much you eat. Having a sandwich using a matchbox-sized piece of cheese, grated to make it go further, means a lump of cheese will last all week instead of just a couple of days. Eating two slices of toast for your breakfast with peanut butter will halve the amount you'd spend on breakfast bread if you used to eat four slices of toast.

And it's easy to spend a fortune on takeaway meals and snatched meals in coffee shops and cafés. Far, far cheaper to make a quick stir-fry when you get home, and carry nuts or apples to tide you over when you are hungry while out and about.

So, don't believe that you can't afford to eat healthily – it probably won't cost you any more. And what about the price of ill health caused by being overweight and undernourished? You can't afford NOT to eat healthily.

Get moving

There is just no getting away from the need for exercise. Our bodies are not designed to slump on the couch every evening, after a day spent sitting in front of a computer screen or in a car. Following the 12-week diet plan means you will gradually get more active.

If you haven't done much exercise for a long time, don't worry. We're not about to ask you to run a marathon in the first month of the programme – or even in the last month for that matter! The aim during the first four weeks of the plan is just to get used to moving again. It's to get your joints freed up, start enjoying the feeling of increased mobility in your joints, and begin to feel hopeful about your body's ability to get in shape once you let it get on with the job. There are two things we want you to do. The first thing is to get walking. If possible, buy or borrow a pedometer and aim to walk 10,000 steps a day. 10,000 steps may sound like a lot, but every step you take soon adds up. For example, if you normally take the bus to work, try getting off a stop early and walk home from there. If you normally sit at your desk at lunchtime, make a point of getting out and about instead – walk around the block for 15 minutes. You'll feel better for the fresh air too.

The second thing we want you to do every day is the range of stretching exercises on pages 60–61. Think of when would be a good time – first thing in the morning when you get out of bed? Last thing at night before you hop in the sack? Once the kids are packed off to school? Only you know when suits you best, but choose a time that you can maintain, consistently. These range of movement exercises are going to be part of your everyday life now.

Wear loose clothing, and before you begin, stand with your arms hanging at your sides. Plant your feet firmly and evenly on the ground. Imagine a string pulling up from the crown of your head. Pull your shoulders up to your ears, then roll them backwards and down. Pull in your stomach muscles, so you feel a tight band from your waist down to your pubic bone. Can you feel your body stretching out, with your backbone coming into alignment? Experiment with tightening muscles and changing the position of your shoulders, hips and legs until you are aligned.

Now you're ready for the stretching exercises on pages 60–61. Do each of the exercises once, but if you are feeling good, repeat the full routine a couple more times. The right way to complete these exercises is slowly and in a relaxed way. You should stretch gently until you feel some mild resistance. This is all about taking pleasure in your body – if you feel any pain it is your body telling you to back off slightly. Move through each position as fully as you can breathing slowly and naturally throughout.

Your daily stretching routine

1. ROTATING NECK

Turn your head slowly to one side and then to the other as far as you can, looking over your shoulder each time.

2. TILTING NECK

Without lifting your shoulders, tilt your head over to one side, as if you were trying to touch your ear to your shoulder. Repeat on the other side.

3. TILTING NECK FORWARDS AND BACKWARDS

Move your head forwards and then backwards, with the top of your head leading the way.

4. STRETCHING BACK, ARMS AND HANDS

Link your hands together with your fingers interlaced. Turn your palms outwards, curve your back and stretch your arms forwards in line with your shoulders.

5. STRETCHING SHOULDERS

Put your right hand on the bent elbow of your left arm and push the elbow gently across in front of the body so your left hand goes over your right shoulder. Repeat on the other side.

6. STRETCHING UPPER BODY

With your hands on your hips, lift at your waist (can you feel yourself getting taller and thinner?), then twist first to the left and then to the right.

7. STRETCHING WAIST

Keeping your hips level, lift your left arm over your head, then bend sideways to the right at the waist, reaching downwards with your left hand. Repeat on the other side.

8. BENDING SPINE

Standing up straight, start to bend forwards leading with the crown of your head and keeping your chin as close to your chest as possible. Visualize each bone in your spine bending forward, one by one. Keep bending over, pulling in your tummy. Relax your shoulders and let your hands hang down towards the floor.

9. STRETCHING LEGS

Stand with your feet about 1m apart. Place your hands on your hips, and with your feet pointing forwards, bend one knee and lean to that side, stretching out the other leg. Repeat on the other side.

10. BENDING LEGS

Stand with your feet about 1m apart with your hands on your hips. Pull in your tummy and slowly bend both knees to lower your bottom towards the floor.

Start doing this range of flexibility exercises every day and they will soon become second nature.

THOUGHT FOR THE WEEK

'When it comes to fitness, small things make a difference. Just get your body moving! Look for opportunities in your day to move more – walk to the shops, take the stairs and do your daily range of movement exercises.' DR BEN

Week 1 2 3 4

Start the week

It's time for that weekly appointment with yourself. Hop on the scales and get out your tape measure to see the results of your first week on the plan. Write down the weight you were last week, and then jot down your weight today. Do the same with your body measurements. If you've been sticking to the rules, you should have lost 1–2lbs.

Look back at the rules on page 47 so you remember what you've got to continue doing this week.

We hope the first week has gone well, and you managed to make changes to your eating habits. Cutting out food and drink that is processed, high in sugar or fat gets rid of empty calories that are not giving you many nutrients. And increasing the amount of fruit, vegetables and wholegrain cereals will be giving you a vitamin and mineral boost. Now you've made a start, you can do a bit of fine-tuning to your particular needs.

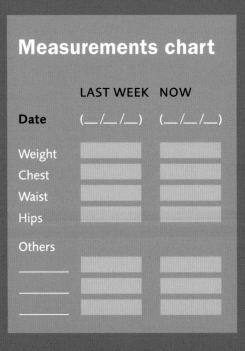

Measurements chart

	LAST WEEK	NOW
Date	(__ /__ /__)	(__ /__ /__)
Weight		
Chest		
Waist		
Hips		
Others		
_____		
_____		
_____		

Let's get personal

If you came to our clinic, or were featured in *The Diet Doctors: Inside and Out*, you'd get our personal attention. We'd develop an eating and exercise plan specifically for you, taking into account your particular health needs and abilities to exercise. It would be based on the 12-week diet plan included in this book, but it would be tweaked and modified to meet your needs.

Although we can't see you face-to-face, we want to try and make the 12-week diet plan as personal to you as possible. Whatever your specific needs, nothing alters the fact that you will only become healthier if you eat well and exercise more, so the basic plan holds for everyone. But what we suggest is you adapt your diet to fit the appearance and health issues you have already identified.

The tables in the appendix on pages 210–216 suggest foods to choose or avoid to help your appearance and health.

'Your body is not working against you – it's desperate to be healthy.' DR BEN

'Help! I feel rubbish'

You may find that during the first week or so of new eating and exercising habits, you don't feel at your best. Don't panic, it'll get better! This is probably because your body has not had enough time to adjust, and it's still a bit early to start feeling the benefits. Your body may be grumbling and complaining, just as children do when they're asked to do something a bit different. Don't worry about it. Just stay with it.

One reason why you may feel so horrible is if you've cut back on cola drinks, tea or coffee. They all contain caffeine or caffeine-like substances. As well as perking you up and getting you going when you're feeling sluggish, caffeine can also affect your heart rate and your brain. Your body will be used to its regular daily caffeine shots. Stopping them is a bit like going cold turkey – you might get headaches and feel lethargic and generally grotty. Try to ease your discomfort in these early days by cutting down slowly on the caffeine, and drinking lots of water or herbal tea.

Remember that your body *will* readjust – and *then* you will start feeling better than before. Too much caffeine is often responsible for insistent nagging headaches, palpitations and sleeping difficulties – and that's without thinking about the effect of all those calories included in a sugary fizzy drink, milky tea or creamy latte. One of the contributors to *The Diet Doctors: Inside and Out* reported in the first week that her head felt like it was going to explode, probably because she'd stopped the 10 cups of sweet tea she had each day. But by the following week she felt like a new woman, and after 12 weeks she'd dropped two dress sizes and lost 9 inches from her waist.

Another reason why you might not feel good is the adjustment to eating less. If you are overweight, then your body has been used to eating more than it needed, and happily tucked away all that extra energy into fat. If you are sticking to the eating plan, you are likely to be eating substantial meals, but with a lower overall calorie intake, so your body is having to get used to burning up that extra fat instead of piling it on – a bit of an adjustment. Eating less sugar also means a readjustment in levels of the hormone, insulin. If part of the grotty feeling is due to hunger, then there is a simple solution – have a snack. No, we don't mean the kind of snack you may be used to (packet of crisps, muffin, chocolate bar). We mean a few nuts (NOT salted peanuts, but nuts such as brazils, walnuts or almonds) ... or a piece of fruit ... or a little box of raisins ... or a cube or two of feta cheese ... or a low-fat yoghurt ... See, there are plenty of ways of having a snack that will stop the hunger pangs but still keep you on track. In fact,

I am *absolutely insists* that her patients have two small snacks a day! So don't try so hard to cut back on food that you make yourself feel hungry.

That grotty feeling could be because you're a bit dehydrated. Remember that most food contains a lot of water. If you are eating less, you will also be taking in less water. This can make you feel tired and headachy, and can make you constipated. So if you're not eating the water, then you need to be drinking it! Keep drinking water throughout the day and it will help you feel better. It's also easy to think you're hungry when actually you're thirsty – again, drinking more will help.

Posture perfect

Now that you are in the second week of the plan, you should have lost a few pounds. But regardless of how much weight you have lost, you will have a much slimmer appearance if you have good posture. Even more importantly, good posture reduces the risk of backache and other problems with joints and muscles. So what's your posture like? When you checked out your appearance (see page 9), what did you score in the posture section? If it was less than a perfect score, read on to find out Dr Ben's top tips for perfect posture.

'When it comes to standing, try to keep weight evenly distributed. Your hips should be level, and so should your shoulders. It's very common to see women walking along with one shoulder higher than the other. I think the fashion for very large bags hasn't helped – it wouldn't be so bad if the bag was large but empty, but women seem to see large bags as things that just have to be filled! My advice would be to leave the extra make-up and clobber at home, so that the bag is light. If it's a shoulder bag, regularly swap the sides that it's carried on, so that your body is not always distorted on one side. And most importantly, try to make sure that you don't pull one shoulder up to try and compensate for the weight of the bag.' **DR BEN**

Ideally, shoes should have a low heel. High heels might make your legs look great, but they throw your backbone out of alignment so can cause problems. If you do wear high heels, make sure that you regularly use low heels too, so that your body has a chance to recover.

Stand tall. Imagine that you are looking over the heads of a crowd, or picture a string tied to the crown of your head and pulling you up. Feel the way that your tummy gets flatter, just from this simple action. Make sure that you don't pull up your shoulders, though. They need to be kept pulled down. Imagine that your shoulders are big wings, and you are trying to push the bottom tips into your back jeans pockets – no more round shoulders!

Week 1 2 **3** 4

Start the week

You're half way through the first stage of the plan already. Jump on the scales and dig out your tape measure to check out your progress. Write down the weight you were last week, and record today's weight. Your weight should be down another pound or two. Remind yourself of the rules by looking back to page 47, then you'll be ready to get going again this week.

If you've not lost any weight or inches yet go back to your food diary to see if any choices you've made have been hindering your progress. Are you following Pam's portion rules for example? How are you getting on with building up to your 10,000 steps a day? Could you walk the kids to school, for example, instead of drive? Are you still fitting in your daily stretching routine? If you're finding it hard, is there another time of day that would be easier to stick to?

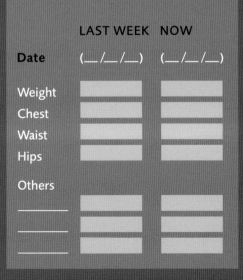

Measurements chart

	LAST WEEK	NOW
Date	(__/__/__)	(__/__/__)
Weight		
Chest		
Waist		
Hips		
Others		
_____		
_____		
_____		

Skin deep

When you assessed your appearance on page 8, did you notice any problems with your skin? As your body is completely wrapped in skin, it's not a surprise that it can easily show when you are not eating enough of the right nutrients. Changes in the skin can also reflect problems elsewhere in the body.

Spotty skin is something we often see in overweight people. If you are heavy, you will know that it's hard work moving your body around, and you might find that you often get hot and sweaty. This can block skin pores and provides ideal conditions for bacteria on the skin to flourish. The result? Oily skin and acne. If this sounds like you, then make sure that you avoid fried and fatty food, and choose shellfish or turkey instead, to give a zinc boost. Eggs, onion and garlic are also good for blemished skin. Make sure you get plenty of water to drink – aim for at least eight glasses a day.

Dry and itchy skin is often a sign of inflammation. It might be a reaction to something you are eating or drinking, or be caused by contact with a particular perfume, washing powder or something else that irritates your skin. Try to work out what is causing the problem and avoid it in the future, but this is usually easier said than done. Changes in your diet may help. Make sure that you are eating at least five portions of fruit and vegetables a day. Cut back on meat and other sources of saturated fats, but increase the amount of fish and seeds you eat each day, to boost unsaturated fats.

Eating regular nutritious meals, cutting out foods that are low in vitamins and losing weight will improve your health on the inside, and you will begin to see improvements in your complexion on the outside.

THOUGHT FOR THE WEEK

'Take a mature and adult attitude to your health and stop resenting what you have to do to keep your body healthy and gorgeous.' PAM

When it comes to sitting, try to use an upright chair with a firm seat, and keep your shoulders down and neck muscles relaxed. When working at a desk, people often sit all hunched up, but this can make the muscles shorten, cause pain across the shoulders and lead to headaches. It is important to stretch out the front of the neck and the shoulder. A good way to do this is standing in an open doorway with your hands at shoulder height and forearms pressed into the door frame. Gently lean forward and feel all the tension drain away.

When you're on the phone, don't lean your head to one side to trap the handset between head and shoulder so your hands are free as this can lead to shoulder and neck problems. And if you have to carry something heavy, make sure that the weight is as evenly distributed as possible. So don't carry toddlers on one hip all the time!

'Never, ever, underestimate the benefits of good posture.' DR BEN

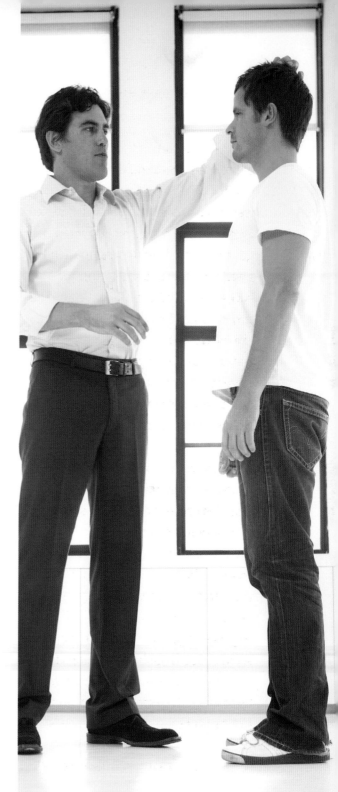

Get into the groove

One of the easiest ways to lose weight is to stick to fixed meal times and snacks. We recommend that you eat five times a day – three meals and two small snacks. If you've been on lots of diets and if the word 'diet' means you expect to be hungry, then the idea of eating five times a day might seem a bit worrying to you. But we don't want you to eat more food, just spread it out evenly through the day. This means that you eat when you're hungry and you use up what you eat as you go along – no storing up of any excess to add to the fat reserves you've already got. Give it a try and see if it helps you. This is what we recommend.

▶ Make sure that you eat breakfast as early as possible in the morning.

▶ Have a healthy snack mid-morning.

▶ Eat lunch around 1 o'clock if you can.

▶ In the afternoon, have another snack (NOT a chocolate bar!) when you feel your energy levels dip – probably around 4 o'clock.

▶ Make sure you eat your last meal of the day at least three hours before you go to bed.

With this pattern, when you wake up you will be hungry and ready for breakfast. If you can't face breakfast, try eating your evening meal a few hours earlier. And if your timetable makes that impossible, switch round your meals so that lunch becomes your main meal and you have a lighter meal in the evening, well before you go to bed. Once you've succeeded in eating less in the evening, you should find that eating breakfast becomes one of life's pleasures, as well as kick-starting your body for the day.

'Help! I'm comfort eating'

Most people eat for a whole host of reasons, and hunger is not always top of the list – emotions such as boredom, stress, frustration, anger, tiredness, annoyance, depression, nervousness, jealousy, guilt, happiness and sadness can all make you hit the biscuit tin or the chocolate counter of the newsagents, big time. Of course, it's perfectly normal to eat for pleasure, as well as just to satisfy hunger. But a problem can arise if the balance is skewed.

'I feel strongly about this. Many people use food as a comfort. It's not usually hunger (in the stomach) that drives people to eat more than they need, it's their appetite. They just want to eat. Try eating well and regularly, and it will help you cut down on the emotional eating. Once you realize you've got lots more energy and feel better, then you'll gradually change too. Listen to your stomach and not your head and you'll never be overweight. Though it seems as though we have endless reasons to eat, there is only one reason why we really need food – for energy!' **PAM**

Look back at the food diary you kept and see what you wrote about your mood each time you ate. How many times did you eat for a reason other than hunger? Identify your problem times and foods, and what triggers your emotional eating. Cut out emotional eating, and eat only when you're genuinely hungry, and you will find your excessive weight starts dropping off.

Banish binges

Many people occasionally overeat and end up feeling full and bloated, but this is actually quite different from a binge-eating disorder. This is when people feel like they've lost control, and eat large quantities of food, very quickly, within a short space of time, even if they're not hungry. Afterwards, they can feel ashamed, disgusted or depressed about all they've eaten.

Extreme emotions, such as feeling sad, angry, worried, anxious or bored can prompt binges. People with a binge-eating disorder are often depressed, though it's not clear if the depression causes the eating problem or vice versa. Although it's mainly a psychological problem, binges can cause huge surges in levels of the hormone insulin, followed by a rapid drop in blood sugar, prompting more eating. If you fit this pattern, with binge episodes at least twice a week for six months or more, then you should discuss it with your GP to help to sort out the problem.

The eating pattern we advise – three meals and two healthy snacks a day, with no more than three or four hours between them – helps because it stops you feeling excessively hungry. Try not to eat outside of the planned meals and snacks, but if you do have a binge, don't miss out any of the meals or snacks to make up for it as it can make the binges worse. Always make time to eat regularly, even if you are busy. Keeping a food diary will help you plan when and what to eat.

When you're shopping for food, don't buy large quantities of any of the foods you might binge on, and make sure you're well stocked up on food that is not a problem for you. When you're cooking, don't taste the food as you go along, as this can also trigger binges.

Never eat standing up, or in the bedroom. Try not to eat when you're watching the television, instead always sit down at a table and use a knife and fork. When you've finished your meal, clear things away, then do something else away from the eating area.

Vitamins and minerals for vitality

Have you noticed how often some foods, such as green leafy vegetables and colourful fruit and veg, are mentioned as sources of different vitamins and minerals, whilst crisps, sweets, croissants, white bread and chocolate are never mentioned at all?

This is because refined foods tend to have very little nutritional value. Look back at the food diary you kept before you started on the 12-week diet plan. Do you think you were eating enough foods containing vitamins and minerals? If not, this could explain some of your tiredness, headaches and other signs of poor health.

We check the vitamin and mineral levels in the blood of all the people we feature on *The Diet Doctors: Inside and Out*, and what we find is often really shocking. Many people are eating all day, far more food than they need, but they're short of the vitamins and minerals that are vital for a healthy body. It could be the same for you.

Following the 12-week plan means that you will get all the nutrients you need for health. If, however, you have been eating a very poor diet for some time, you may actually be suffering from a severe vitamin or mineral deficiency which needs to be supplemented to boost your diet and get your levels back to normal.

The vitamins and minerals listed over the page are the most common deficiencies that we see in our clinics. If you think you may be deficient in one or more of them, you should consider seeing a nutritionist. They can take and test blood samples, and advise if you should be taking any supplements alongside the 12-week plan.

THOUGHT FOR THE WEEK

'If you're overweight, chances are you're unhealthy.' DR SAMINA

'Many people are overfed yet undernourished. There are plenty of thin people who have extremely poor diets – weight isn't the only issue.' PAM

Common deficiencies

B GROUP VITAMINS

The B vitamins are found in food sources such as lean meats, brewer's yeast, wholegrains and vegetable proteins, such as beans. Although they are individually distinct from each other, the B vitamins tend to work together and are closely interrelated. This is why, if supplementing, a B complex is generally a better option than individual B vitamins.

The B vitamins are necessary for energy production, metabolism and for the nervous system. Symptoms of deficiencies include mouth, tongue or lip sores, depression, irritability, weakness, fatigue, poor concentration, and numbness and tingling in the hands and feet. Binge drinkers, alcoholics, women taking the contraceptive pill long term, and those on a junk food diet are more at risk of deficiency.

CALCIUM

Calcium is hugely important for the health of bones, teeth, nerves, muscles, skin and hair. The body strives to keep the calcium levels steady in the blood and will do so at the expense of your bones if dietary intake is low. You need sufficient calcium (with vitamin D) to attain and maintain peak bone mass (strong bones) and prevent osteoporosis later in life. Tooth damage or decay, muscle cramps and brittle or soft bones are all signs that you may be deficient. Make sure you include plenty of calcium-rich foods in your diet, such as dairy products, green leafy vegetables, fish where the bones are eaten (such as sardines and tinned salmon), nuts, seeds and beans, such as soya. Menopausal women may benefit from supplementation.

CHROMIUM

Chromium is vital to the function of insulin and is required by most cells for uptake of glucose. Deficiency is quite common in people eating a huge amount of simple sugars – symptoms include energy slumps, dizziness and mood swings – so if this sounds like you, consider getting your levels tested.

IRON

Iron is hugely important and woman can become quite deficient if they have heavy periods and a low dietary intake. Symptoms include tiredness, brittle, ridged nails, depression and muscle weakness. In the National Diet and Nutrition Survey 8% of women tested had iron deficiency anaemia, and 11% of women had low iron stores (ferritin levels). However, you mustn't take a supplement unless you have been tested as too much iron can cause problems too.

MAGNESIUM

Irritability, weight loss, tiredness, difficulty sleeping, muscle twitching, problems with memory, and confusion are all symptoms of magnesium deficiency. Increase magnesium-rich foods to your diet, such as legumes, nuts and seeds, fruits and vegetables, wholegrains and soy products, and consider getting your magnesium levels checked by a nutritionist.

SELENIUM

Selenium supports many functions in the body, including making antioxidant enzymes, strengthening immunity, maintaining thyroid health and helping fertility. Signs of a deficiency include tiredness, frequent infections, poor wound healing and premature ageing. Plant foods, such as vegetables and grains, fish, shellfish, red meat, brewer's yeast and wheatgerm are the most common dietary sources.

VITAMIN C

If you have noticed inflamed bleeding gums, dry splitting hair, easy bruising, fatigue, and weight gain it could be that you are getting too little vitamin C in your diet. In the National Nutrition Survey 5% of men and 3% of women had a vitamin C deficiency. If taking a vitamin C supplement, don't have more than 500mg per day without professional advice.

ZINC

Poor appetite, hair problems, numerous infections and slow wound healing are just some signs of zinc deficiency. However individual zinc supplementation above the RDA needs professional nutritional advice since too much zinc at one time will not be well absorbed and can actually increase bacterial infections.

Week 1 2 3 **4**

Start the week

You're about to start the last week of the first part of the plan. So get out the scales and tape measure again to see how you are getting on. Like last week your weight should be 1–2lbs down from last week's weight. Start the week well by reminding yourself of the rules (page 47).

Measurements chart

	LAST WEEK (__/__/__)	NOW (__/__/__)
Date		
Weight		
Chest		
Waist		
Hips		
Others		
_____		
_____		
_____		

Label lingo

Food labelling has been introduced so that you can see what's in the food that you are buying. To make the food look appealing days after it's been prepared, and to keep it fresh enough to eat, manufacturers have to add preservatives, colouring and other additives. They might have added salt to boost flavour and included trans fats (also called hydrogenated fats on the label) to give long shelf-life. But excess salt makes blood pressure rise, and trans fats increase the risk of heart disease (see page 105), while studies have shown that additives and preservatives can lead to disruptive and aggressive behaviour in children. Cooking from simple and fresh ingredients avoids these unwanted extras. But even if you decide to shun the ready meal aisle in the supermarket, what's in all the other food that you can't live without? The trick is to learn how to read the label. The simplest system of food labelling is based on traffic lights: red, amber and green to indicate high, medium and low levels of calories, fat, sugar and salt in 100g of the food. This means that you can easily compare different foods, and choose the one with the most green lights. For example, if you are browsing the shelf for a quick sandwich during your lunch break, you might choose the poached salmon and cucumber in wholegrain bread with its four green lights, rather than the egg, bacon and sausage sandwich in white bread with warning lights on the label.

Unfortunately, not all manufacturers or supermarkets have adopted the simple traffic light system. Many big manufacturers are using a system based on guideline daily amounts for calories, fats, sugars and salts – the advised limit that the average person should eat each day. The panel shows the proportion of this daily limit you would have if you ate a standard-sized serving of the food. You need to look for foods with a low percentage in these panels. Sometimes manufacturers try to disguise the amount of salt by listing the amount of sodium. Sodium is one of the constituents of salt, so you need to multiply the amount of sodium by 2.4 to find out the equivalent amount of salt. 5g of sugar is the equivalent of a teaspoon. There's sugar in a surprising number of foods. Did you realize that there can be 5 teaspoons of sugar in a bowl of tomato soup?

As well as the information on the front of the packaging, most food packets and tins contain a panel of information on the back giving a more detailed breakdown of what's inside, and a list of all the ingredients, starting with the main one.

So after you've read the label, what should you do? First of all, think about the size of the portion that the manufacturer has used for the calculations. Is it realistic? If you were going to eat the whole ready meal yourself when the labelling refers to only half the packet, you would automatically be eating twice as many calories, twice as much fat, twice as much sugar and twice as much salt as suggested on the front of the packet – not necessarily a good idea! As you will know by now, the only way to lose weight is to eat fewer calories each day than your body needs. So avoiding foods that are high in calories will make it easier for you to achieve your goals. A woman should not usually eat more than 2000 calories a day, and a man not more than 2500 calories a day. If you eat more than these amounts, you are likely to put on weight, while eating less should result in weight loss.

We suggest that you avoid food that's high in fat. Fat packs in twice as many calories per 100g than protein or sugar, so keeping away from foods containing lots of fat will help reduce the amount of calories you eat. If there is fat in the food, it is better if it is unsaturated, which usually means it is from vegetable or fish sources. To help your heart and blood vessels stay healthy, avoid foods that are high in saturated fats. And steer clear of foods that contain trans or hydrogenated fats.

Avoid food that includes a lot of salt – remember that the recommended daily limit for adults is 6g from all the food that is eaten. If you have a meal containing 4g on its own, then you are very likely to exceed the healthy level by the time you have eaten other meals.

WHAT'S THE LIMIT?

Daily maximum amounts for the average person

	MAN	WOMAN
Calories	2000	2500
Sugar	50g	62g
Fat	70g	100g
Salt	6g	6g
Sodium	2.5g	2.5g

Wise up to the tricks used in food labelling. Remember that advertising a food as sugar-free doesn't mean it isn't high in fat, and conversely, a food that is advertised as low-fat could well be loaded with sugar. Check out the labels to find out. If a food is labelled '90 per cent fat-free', it doesn't necessarily mean it's a good choice. It means that 100g of the food contains 10g of fat. If it was a ready meal that had a portion size of 350g, that means you would eat 35g of fat – half the maximum recommended amount for a woman in a day – just within one part of a single meal.

See how easy it is to overeat, unless you know the label lingo!

Diabetes danger

Diabetes is often mentioned in the newspapers these days. Having diabetes means that your blood sugar is higher than it should be. There are essentially two types. People with type 1 usually have it diagnosed when they are young when their bodies fail to produce adequate amounts of the hormone insulin, making it necessary for them to inject replacement insulin. It's the type 2 diabetes that is the real hot topic as more and more people are developing it, often as a direct result of their unhealthy lifestyles.

The risk of developing type 2 diabetes is particularly high in people who regularly eat more than their body needs and so damage their ability to cope with it all. The outward sign of this is a build up of fat around your middle, known as an apple shaped physique. A waist measurement of more than 32 inches or 81cm in women and 37 inches or 94cm in men may mean you are at particular risk. If you fit this picture, it might be a good idea to visit your GP and get checked out for diabetes with a simple blood test. Your doctor may also check you for raised blood pressure and cholesterol as these symptoms can often occur together in a cluster known as metabolic syndrome.

If you do develop type 2 diabetes the concern is that high blood sugar levels can damage small blood vessels in the eyes – leading to blindness – and in the kidneys so they stop working too. Having diabetes also increases the likelihood of a heart attack or a stroke occurring. Fortunately many people who are diagnosed early can reduce their blood sugar levels by altering their diet and so minimising the damage.

'If you have been eating a lot of sugar, your chromium levels might be low, making it harder for insulin to do its job. Eat lots of food rich in chromium, things like wholegrains, nuts and seeds. Cut down the amount of sugar in tea and coffee. Balance your blood sugar levels by eating regularly, and make sure that you don't skip meals, particularly breakfast. If someone is diagnosed with diabetes, I like to check their vitamin B, C and D levels, and also their levels of magnesium. I often find that they are low in all these essential nutrients. I also check the amounts of fats they are eating, and discuss the importance of cutting back on saturated and trans fats, while boosting their intake of the essential unsaturated omega fats.' **PAM**

'When you have diabetes it is important to exercise. Exercise will help your body regulate your blood sugar, improve the health of your heart and control your weight. But remember that you have a serious medical condition. You must not exercise to exhaustion or allow your blood sugar level to drop too low. When exercising, drink plenty of water, monitor your blood sugar levels, carry diabetic identification and carry appropriate medication. Check for any cuts or blisters on your feet after training.' **DR BEN**

'Help! How can I stick to the plan when I'm eating out?'

Going out? Don't panic! Eating is often about socializing as well as fuelling up. We're not going to be killjoys and tell you to turn down everything you fancy and stick with a salad. However, it is sensible to think ahead to help you stay on track.

The first thing is to do as Pam does and make sure you don't nibble on the bread that often arrives with the first round of drinks. You'll enjoy your main meal more and avoid unnecessary calories. Remember it's always possible to choose two starters instead of a starter and a main meal, to keep the portion size down. Steer clear of huge pasta dishes, particularly those with cheesy sauces, as they are likely to be very high in calories without a great deal of beneficial nutrients. Paté, fried food and meat served in heavy sauces are also best avoided.

A good choice to start with would be something like a soup or salad (without dressing or served separately so you can add the amount you want), followed by fish or grilled meat. You can control portion sizes by simply leaving some of the potatoes, chips or rice accompanying your meal. When it comes to desserts, choose something fruity and pass on the cream or ice cream. If you are desperate for the chocolate gateau or crème caramel, have what you fancy but why not share it with someone else, to keep the portion size down?

At buffets, decide in advance what is a reasonable amount to eat, and then stick to it – remember, lots of little tasty morsels soon add up to a rather large amount. Choose the low-fat options, like salmon or vegetable sticks with a dip, rather than deep-fried cheese wedges or salami. Move away from the buffet when you've had what you'd planned to have.

Make sure you drink water with your meal. Having a regular sip of water ensures that you eat slowly enough for your mind to register that you are getting full.

HOW DOES DR SAMINA DO IT?

'I start the day with freshly squeezed orange juice then have some fat-free organic yoghurt with fresh fruit, such as melon, mango or blueberries, depending on what's in the fridge. I often have a couple of slices of toast with butter and home-made jam or mashed avocado. My partner introduced me to this – we always have a range of avocados in the house, from rock solid to nice and squidgy. I have fresh coffee with semi-skimmed milk but no sugar.

'I leave for work at around 7.30–8.00, and it takes 30–45 minutes. I park about 10 minutes from the surgery, so I always get a walk, usually carrying large bundles of patient notes (good toning exercise!). Mid-morning, I have a cup of coffee or tea and a piece of fruit or a biscuit.

'Lunch is usually between 1 and 2 o'clock. I either take in something from home – a salad or sandwich with tuna, chicken, smoked salmon or beef – or I fetch soup or a sandwich from the organic café nearby. I often have a yoghurt or fruit as well.

'I leave work anytime between 6pm and 9pm. I usually have a few nuts or olives with a small glass of wine while cooking dinner. Once a week, this is a curry dish of meat, fish or vegetables. My father comes from Pakistan and he's a good cook, as well as a GP and former heart surgeon, so he's taught me how to cook healthy curries. Otherwise, it's grilled fish, roast chicken or something simple with fresh vegetables or salad.

'If we go out to eat, I usually choose shellfish or fish, but sometimes I go for the steak and French fries option. If it's really late by the time I get home, I'll have something quick and light, like smoked salmon on toast with a salad, instead of a full dinner. I really hate the feeling of going to bed too full, but I can't sleep if I'm too hungry either.

'Apart from my walk to and from the car each day, I struggle to fit in other exercise during the week, but I make sure that I fit in something at the weekend. Usually I prefer to be outside, walking or horse-riding, which is totally de-stressing after a week indoors.'

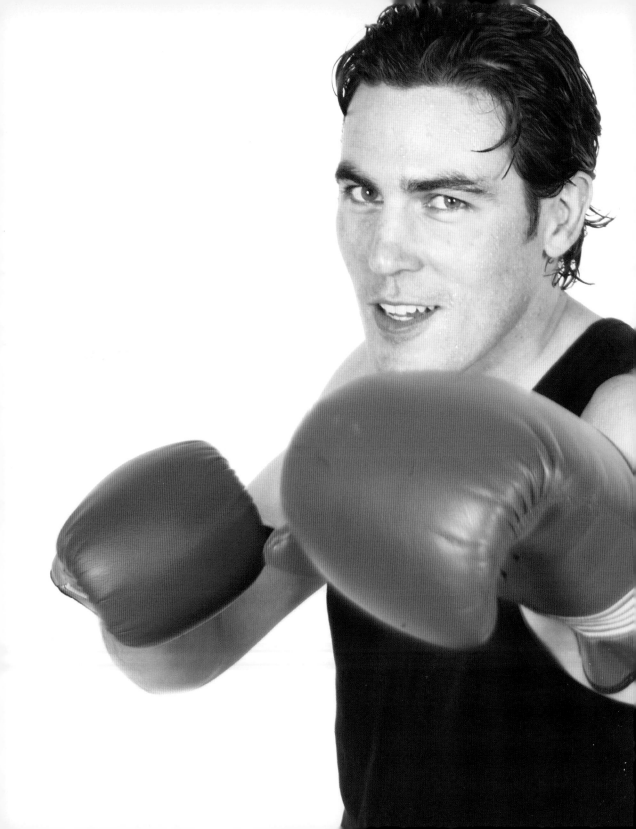

CHAPTER 4

Weeks 5–8

What's going to happen this month?

During the last few weeks you've been shifting your eating patterns. Look back and think about the things that worked well, and any pitfalls. How can you overcome any difficulties? For example, if you struggle to fit in your daily stretching exercises, could you get up earlier?

It's now time for the second phase of the plan. This month, we want you to build on the rules from weeks 1–4. This means continuing with the three meals and two healthy snacks a day (remember that each one needs to include a little protein) and eating five portions of fruit and veg a day.

This month we'd like you to eat a wider variety of nutritious foods. We now want you to eat more fish – at least two portions a week, one of which should be oily fish, such as salmon, mackerel or sardines.

You still need to keep an eye on your portion sizes and cut back on your high-fat, high-sugar intake. Make sure you have no more than one portion a week.

The same rules apply to water and alcohol – remember, if you must have alcohol when socializing, limit yourself to no more than one small drink a day (such as a small 125ml glass of wine or a small bottle of beer).

We want you to keep going with your Daily Stretching Routine and walking, but now we need you to start exercising your heart and lungs as well. Exercising your heart and lungs won't just make you fitter and flood your body with natural feel-good chemicals for a healthy high. It will also help you burn fat faster and avoid the weight loss plateau that often happens a month or so into a diet. Aim for at least three cardio sessions a week. Don't worry if you hate the gym as we'll get you moving in other ways (see page 102).

Finally, keep going with your food and mood diary and stick to your weekly appointment to weigh and measure your progress. Following the second part of the 12-week diet plan should result in a further 4–8lbs weight loss.

The rules for weeks 5–8

1. Eat three meals and two healthy snacks every day, including a little protein each time

2. Eat five portions of fruit and vegetables every day, day in day out

3. Eat at least two portions of fish a week

4. Eat no more than one portion of high fat, high sugar food a week

5. Make sure that your portion sizes don't creep up

6. Keep drinking water

7. Continue to take a break from alcohol

8. Continue with the Daily Stretching Routine on pages 60–61 every day

9. Aim to walk 10,000 steps a day

10. Start exercising your heart and lungs, aiming for at least three sessions a week

11. Weigh and measure yourself at the start of each week

12. Keep up your food and mood diary

Week 5 6 7 8

Start the week

Before you move onto the second stage of the 12-week diet plan let's take a look at your progress. If you've been sticking to the plan you should have lost 4–8lbs over the last four weeks. Fill in your starting and goal weights in the chart below, then step on the scales, get out your tape measure and fill in your current weight and measurements.

Are you making progress towards your goal? It's great if things are going well for you and you are on track – you can move on to this next stage of the plan feeling pleased with yourself.

Measurements chart

	START	NOW	GOAL
Date	(__/__/__)	(__/__/__)	(__/__/__)
Weight			
Chest			
Waist			
Hips			
Others			
_____			
_____			
_____			

If you have not lost 4lbs, ask yourself if you have followed the plan. Remind yourself what we wanted you to do – cut out food that is high in calories but low in nutrients (takeaways and ready meals, sugary and salty foods, and soft drinks). We wanted you to eat regular meals with sensible-sized portions, and healthy snacks to stop you feeling hungry. Have you done this? Look back at your food diary to see if you can spot any patterns or pitfalls that are holding you back. It might also help you to take the Healthy Eating questionnaire on page 35 again. As you start the next stage of the plan, make sure that you stick to the basic rules given on page 89.

Check your flexibility again, using the test on pages 30–31. Doing the range of stretching exercises each day during the last 4 weeks should have improved your flexibility. You should now be used to moving your body, and be ready for the next stage of the plan.

What's on the menu?

Now you're in the breakfast habit, you might want to increase variety and try out some new morning foods. Can you include at least one of your five portions of fruit and vegetables with your breakfast? Make sure that your breakfast includes some protein (meat, fish, egg, nuts) or dairy produce (milk, low-fat cheese, yoghurt). Cereals and bread should be wholegrain to make sure you get a good helping of vitamins.

Breakfast

IN A RUSH	30g bran flakes or oat clusters with fruit (e.g. a sliced banana, handful of berries, chopped apple), scattering of ground flax seeds and skimmed or semi-skimmed milk
	30g muesli with no added sugar but containing nuts and dried fruit, with added fresh fruit and natural yoghurt
	Porridge made with 30g oats and skimmed or semi-skimmed milk and topped with mixed nuts, seeds and chopped fruit
	Two slices wholegrain toast topped with sliced tomato and smoked salmon
	Two slices wholegrain toast topped with mashed avocado (see recipe on page 162)
	Two Ryvita or slices of rye bread spread with cottage cheese and chopped cucumber
TIME TO COOK	Half a grapefruit, followed by a boiled egg served with two oatcakes
	Omelette made with two eggs, with chopped fresh herbs inside
	Two slices wholegrain toast with small can of baked beans
	Two slices wholegrain toast topped with a slice of ham, grilled tomatoes and grilled mushrooms
SHAKES AND SMOOTHIES (See recipes on pages 160–161)	Kiwi, yoghurt and sesame seed shake
	Yoghurt, flax seed and frozen berry smoothie
	Pineapple and banana shake

Snacks

You might want to continue with the healthy snacks you've been having mid-morning and mid-afternoon during the last few weeks, or you might be ready to try out some new ideas. Make sure that your snack includes a small amount of protein to stop you feeling hungry too soon. You can also use the snack as an opportunity to fit in another fruit or vegetable portion.

NUTS	Five or six unsalted nuts (brazils, pecans, almonds, walnuts, hazelnuts) with a kiwi fruit, apple or a handful of raisins
	An oatcake or crispbread spread with peanut butter or pesto (see recipe on page 162)
DAIRY	Apple with a small piece of feta cheese
	A rice cake spread with no-fat soft cheese
	Small pot of live natural yoghurt with a scattering of chopped dried apricots, dates or figs
FISH	A rice cake or crispbread spread with Dr Samina's tapenade (see recipe on page 163)
	Couple of chunky rings of cucumber topped with smoked salmon
VEGETABLES	Cut-up raw vegetables inside a small wholemeal pitta bread
	Tablespoon of hummus with raw vegetables (cherry tomatoes, carrot sticks, celery, cauliflower florets, strips of red, yellow and green peppers)
	An oatcake spread with mashed avocado or chickpea dip (see recipe on page 163)

'Once you get into the swing of it, preparing delicious, healthy food for you and your family is simple ... and can be cheaper than buying ready-prepared meals.' PAM

Lunches

If you'd like to add a bit more variety and be more adventurous with your lunches, try some of the ideas below. Try to include fish or shellfish regularly, and also pulses or beans. You can also use the salad ideas as toppings or sandwich fillings – but only use one topping, and make sure you use wholegrain or granary bread. Avoid butter or mayo, as they add unnecessary calories. Or follow Dr Ben's approach and use a drizzle of olive oil.

Simple salads

Choose up to five bases and a couple of toppings for a great salad, with a squirt of lemon juice or drop of olive oil, mixed with fresh chopped herbs, as a dressing

BASES	TOPPINGS
Mixed lettuce leaves	Slice of ham
Watercress	Tablespoon of tuna
Chunks of cucumber	Handful of cashew nuts or pine nuts
Sliced tomatoes	Few anchovies
Diced red or yellow peppers	Few sardines from a tin
Cold cooked French beans	Slice of chicken breast
Baby spinach leaves	Slice of smoked salmon
Finely diced red onion	Tablespoon of prawns
Bean sprouts	Slice of lean beef
Grated carrot	Tablespoon of diced feta cheese
Finely sliced red and white cabbage	Tablespoon of cottage cheese
Chopped avocado	Tablespoon of chickpeas
Cauliflower or broccoli florets	Chopped boiled egg

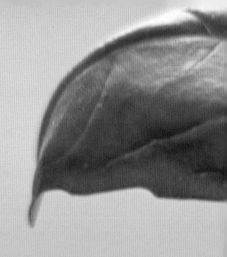

Soup

Soup makes a delicious and nutritious warming lunch. Vegetables used in soups count towards your daily five portions. Buy good quality soup available in the chiller section of the supermarket, or make your own. Soups are cheap and easy to make, particularly if you have a blender that can be used directly in the pan. You can be as inventive as you like with the combinations you use. Follow the recipes included for these soup suggestions starting on page 164, or experiment with your own combinations.

Simple soups

- Roast tomato and basil
- Easy minestrone
- Red lentil, carrot and chilli
- Borlotti bean soup
- Lentil soup with spinach

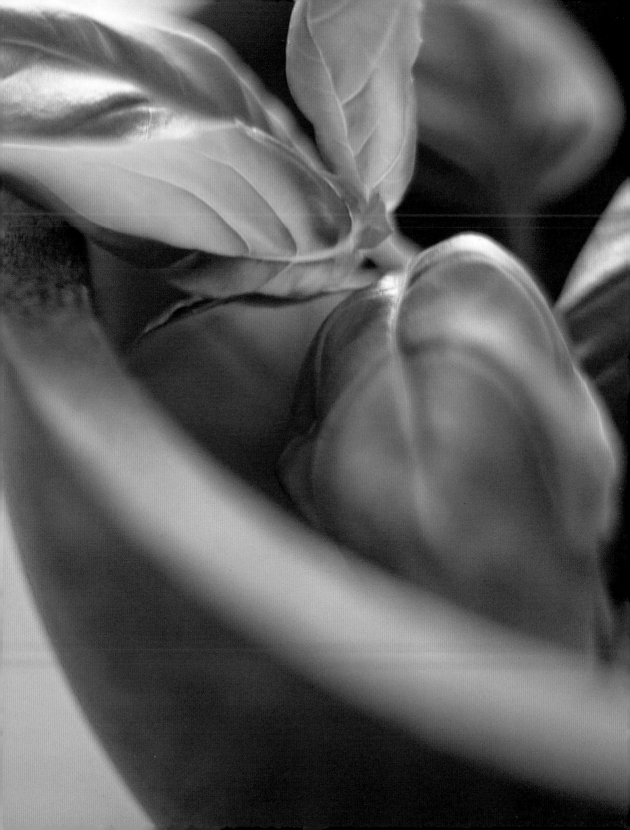

Dinners

If you're happy that your evening meals have become more nutritious and your weight loss is continuing, then it's fine to carry on with what you are doing. But you may also want to introduce some new dinner ideas. We've included some suggestions here, with the recipes starting on page 170. You could also spend some time looking through cookery books and at recipe ideas in magazines – there are masses of meal suggestions to choose from. Remember that you are looking for dinners that include a high proportion of vegetables, with some protein or dairy produce. You can eat up to a third of the meal as potato, rice or pasta, if you are already at the right weight for your height. However, when you want to lose weight, it is better to restrict this food group to a much smaller portion and use the space on your plate for more vegetables – you should be aiming for around half of the meal being vegetables. So if you cook a dinner based on rice or pasta, remember to serve yourself only a small portion. If you are used to having meat with every dinner, it is a good idea to start replacing some of these meals with dinners based on fish.

You can also experiment with vegetarian meals, using beans, pulses, cheese and nuts to provide nutrients in place of meat or fish. Skip ahead to the menu plan for Weeks 9–12 (page 128) if you want some inspiration for vegetarian meals.

During the last few weeks, you should have stopped eating sweets, chocolates, biscuits, ice cream and other high-fat or high-sugar desserts. We want you to continue to give these high-calorie foods a miss, and stick to fruit or yoghurt for dessert, with perhaps the odd square of dark chocolate (70 per cent cocoa) if you are desperate. However, if you are beginning to crave a dessert, look ahead to Weeks 9–12 (page 128) for some ideas for healthy puds.

IN A RUSH

– dinner in around 30 minutes

Coconut chicken

Linguine with smoked salmon

Paella with chicken and prawns

Tuna, rocket and lemon pasta

Halibut with lemon

TIME TO COOK

Lamb goulash

Spicy minced lamb with peas

Lamb tikka

Karahi chicken

Chicken with white beans, tomatoes and olives

Fish pie

Fish curry

'Help! I can't live without…'

Well have it then! We are not trying to make you miserable, so if it is really bothering you, give yourself permission to have whatever you're desperate for. But having said that, think very carefully about the amount you have, and when you have it. For example, if you used to have chocolate on an empty stomach at 4pm, then try and avoid reactivating that pattern. Have the chocolate after a meal instead.

We are assuming that the food you are desperate for is not one on the plan – it seems unlikely that you'd be asking for help if you couldn't live without bananas, beans or broccoli! It's not a problem if you can't live without chocolate, for example, if it's just a single square at the end of your meal, or if you can't live without sliced white bread, as long as you limit yourself to just a slice a day. The problem only arises if you eat a lot of it.

You might find that you are desperate for a food, such as peanuts or biscuits, and once you start eating them you can't stop. These are often called trigger foods. They can lead to binges in some people – see page 73 for more on binge eating. Some people seem to be 'addicted' to certain types of food – usually fatty or sugary. Sugar is known for its addictive qualities, as it can cause a rush of insulin which then rapidly removes sugar from the blood so that you want more bread, biscuits and sugar to fill the gap. You may be part of a family or group of friends that eats lots of sugar so it seems like normal behaviour. Advertising for the food industry can also make it seem part of everyday life to eat these foods. If you think you are 'addicted' to certain foods, then try reducing the amount you have gradually, so that your body doesn't suffer too badly from withdrawal effects.

'If you are eating a food compulsively at home, then make it a rule never to buy it to take home. Limit yourself to single servings when you are out.' PAM

Keep moving

You should now be in the habit of walking 10,000 steps a day and moving your body every day, in a way that makes you feel energized and increases the range of movement in your joints. You need to carry on with the walking and the daily flexibility exercises on pages 60–61 every day during the next four weeks. But now we want you to start working your heart and lungs as well. If they're going to perform well so you can live a long life, they need to be exercised regularly. After all, the heart is a muscle that can be strengthened, and you can improve the functioning of your lungs with practice too. The result will be an improvement in the way that blood is pumped round your body, increasing the amount of oxygen and nutrients, and improving the quality of your body tissues. And as an added bonus – you will look better and feel better.

Exercise that makes your heart beat faster (called cardiovascular exercise) is a great way to improve your mood and has been shown to reduce depression. It helps you sleep better and, because it helps you use up more energy, helps weight loss too. All in all, a very good thing!

So are we going to tell you to get down to the gym and pound away on a treadmill? No – or only if that's the type of cardiovascular exercise that you like. There are lots of different ways to exercise your heart, lungs and blood circulation, and going to a gym is only one of them. What matters is choosing the type of exercise that you find enjoyable. What suits you, your life, your abilities and your pocket will not necessarily be the right thing for someone else. You should aim for three to five 30-minute sessions a week of exercise that raises your heart rate. You might like one activity so much that you do it repeatedly, or you might prefer different types of exercise for each session.

Whatever you do, enjoy it

Whatever kind of cardio exercise you choose it's important that you like it – if the gym is torture for you you'll never stick to it long term! Have a think about what exercise appeals to you most. There are plenty of suggestions below. Are you a sociable person? If so, joining a club, such as a badminton group or a dance class, might work for you. If you prefer time out on your own then cycling or running might be better.

You can start gently with one or two sessions a week, but try to get to three or four sessions a week as soon as you can. Remember, the aim is to raise your heartbeat. For example, a 10-minute gentle stroll is fine this week, but try to ensure that you work up to a 30-minute brisk walk in the next couple of weeks.

CARDIOVASCULAR EXERCISE

Walking	**Rugby**
Line dancing	**Running**
Swimming	**Belly dancing**
Cycling	**Aerobics**
Salsa	**Jogging**
Football	**Ice skating**
Boxing	**Step class**
Rollerblading	**Squash**
Horse riding	**Golf**
Fencing	**Badminton**
Tennis	**Ballroom dancing**
Circuit training	

'If you are overweight, then you are eating too much. It doesn't actually matter if your genes make you susceptible to putting on weight, or that you are small, or that you used to be able to eat more when you were younger than you do now, or when you did more exercise. All that really matters is that you are eating too much – for you – now, period.' PAM

Week 5 6 7 8

Start the week

This week is the half way point. Keep your appointment with yourself to check out your weight and measurements. Record them in the space below so you can see how well you are getting on. You should be aiming to lose around one pound each week. Look back to the rules on page 89 to help you stay on track.

Measurements chart

	LAST WEEK (__/__/__)	NOW (__/__/__)
Date		
Weight		
Chest		
Waist		
Hips		
Others		
_____		
_____		
_____		

The heart of the matter

Your heart is probably the most important muscle in your body, responsible for pumping blood round 24/7, from before birth to the day you die. And heart attacks are the biggest killer in the country. Every two minutes, someone has a heart attack in the UK, which proves fatal for more than 100,000 people each year.

So what does your heart need to be healthy? There are a number of things you can do that can make a very real difference to the health of your heart and blood vessels.

- Lose weight by eating less and exercising more (in a healthy way, as in our 12-week diet plan).
- Reduce the level of cholesterol in your blood by cutting the amount of fat you eat and switching from eating saturated fat in animal products (such as meat, cheese and butter) to unsaturated fat from vegetable sources (like olive oil, sunflower oil, nuts and seeds) or fish (like tuna, salmon and sardines).

- Lower your blood pressure by losing weight, cutting the amount of salt in your diet, increasing the amount of fruit and vegetables, and exercising more.
- Exercise your heart so it gets stronger – exercise also helps with weight loss and lowering blood pressure.
- Stop smoking.

Following the 12-week diet plan will help with the weight loss. But this week, let's spend a little time thinking about why what you eat matters as well.

Food from animal products like meat, cheese and butter contains saturated fats. These tend to be solid at room temperature. Look at the grill pan after you've cooked sausages, bacon or burgers – the liquid fat that comes out of the meat while you're cooking becomes a white solid mass when it cools down. Of course, not all of the fat comes out. You will have eaten a fair amount still trapped inside the meat. In your liver, the saturated fats you ate are turned into another type of fat: cholesterol.

Your body needs some cholesterol, and it is transported around in the blood. However, if there's a lot of cholesterol in your blood, it can get stuck to the inside of blood vessels, making them narrower. Over time, these fatty areas can get bigger, and blood can clot on the damaged area. This makes it difficult for blood to flow through. If the blockage occurs in the blood vessels in heart muscle, you have a heart attack. If the clot blocks the blood vessels supplying the brain, then you have a stroke.

Although strokes and heart attacks usually happen to older people, the damage to the blood vessels can start years before and gets worse if you continue to eat foods that lead to high cholesterol levels. Changing your diet stops this process and can start undoing the damage.

So what should you do if you want to stop the cholesterol rot? Our 12-week diet plan will help. Our plan cuts down on the amount of saturated fat you are eating while boosting the amount of healthy unsaturated fats that tend to be oils at room temperature. Unsaturated fats, such as the essential omega oils found in nuts, seeds and fish, help protect blood vessels. We also ask you to eat foods like beans, lentils, chickpeas and oats that contain soluble fibre. This lowers the amount of bad cholesterol whilst increasing the amount of 'good' cholesterol.

When blood vessels become narrower with stiffer walls, it's harder for the blood to be pumped through and this increases blood pressure. The heart has to work harder if blood pressure is high, and this can damage it. You can reduce your blood pressure by eating less salt, eating more fruit and vegetables, and being more active.

We've not discussed smoking at all in the 12-week diet plan. But if you do smoke, think long and hard about what you are doing to your body. Smokers are much more likely than non-smokers to have a heart attack or stroke, as well as other life-threatening diseases like cancer.

'Help! I'm too busy to cook'

Whether it's because of a whirling social life, the demands of family life or the pressures of work, we all know that cooking can sometimes feel like one thing too many. Sometimes, you just want to drop when you get in and have your dinner taken care of – it's not always the effort involved in the cooking itself that's a problem; it's thinking what to have and then having the ingredients available. That's when you might be tempted to reach for the phone and have a takeaway delivered. So what should you choose to limit the damage you could do to your eating plan?

Takeaway pizzas are not a good choice as they tend to be loaded with calories and saturated fat from all the cheese. If you do have a pizza, it's better to steer clear of those topped with processed meats such as sausage, pepperoni and ham, and definitely no extra cheese – go for reduced-fat cheese if it's available and choose a topping that is mainly vegetables (fresh tomato, mushrooms, sweetcorn) or up the protein by

choosing a fish topping (tuna, anchovies, salmon) and at least you will be getting some useful vitamins.

If it's an Indian takeaway you fancy, choose dry dishes such as tandoori chicken or fish, and vegetable dishes such as spinach and lentils, avoiding sauces which can be high in fat and salt. Plain pilau rice is a good choice, as you may be less tempted to eat a large portion than with naan bread and chapatti. Think twice before choosing samosas and other fried items like onion bhajis as they can be very high in calories.

Chinese food is probably not a good choice if you've got high blood pressure, as it's often very high in salt (or other forms of sodium) as well as fats. Steer clear if you can, but if you can't, go for steamed or stir-fried dishes. And why not share one portion of rice between two?

If you've no time to cook, you might just grab a burger on the way home.

If you do find yourself in a burger bar, remember that you *don't* have to choose the burger; you could choose a salad (without dressing which can bump up the calories enormously). If you desperately want a burger, go for a small plain one in a wholemeal bun, and have it with a salad and fruit juice. Better still might be to walk past the burger bar and go to the chippie instead. Choose a piece of fish, but don't eat the batter, and go light on the chips – you could have just the fish, or share a small portion of chips. Don't worry about the tomato ketchup, though, as it's actually quite nutritious!

Have you thought of alternatives to takeaways if you feel too pressurized to cook? Have a look at how Dr Ben copes (on page 147) and check out his Arabic feast on page 200. You might also want to start planning ahead so that you've got something ready for when you are too busy to cook – again, Dr Ben takes this approach so he can eat as soon as he gets home from work.

'I'm often so hungry when I get home from work that I've just *had* to work out a way of eating good healthy nutritious food without delay – I definitely feel better now that I've got fast food sorted, without having to resort to eating rubbish.' **DR BEN**

'We live in an age when so many of us are obsessed with how we look on the outside. If only we paid a little more attention to what's going on in the inside.' **DR SAMINA**

Week 5 6 **7** 8

Start the week

What is your weight now? Hop on the scales and record your weight then get out your tape measure and record your body measurements as well. If your weight loss is beginning to slow down, don't worry. We've got some suggestions for you this week. But first of all, read the rules again to make sure that you are not letting things slip!

Measurements chart

	LAST WEEK	NOW
Date	(__ /__ /__)	(__ /__ /__)
Weight		
Chest		
Waist		
Hips		
Others		
_____		
_____		
_____		

Gut wrenching

Irritable bowel syndrome (IBS) affects nearly two in ten people in the UK. Symptoms include constipation, diarrhoea, bloating, cramping and flatulence. The pain can be intense. Sometimes it's possible to identify trigger foods, but erratic eating may also bring on attacks, when periods of insufficient food intake alternate with bingeing on large quantities.

In addition to eating regularly, you can help ease symptoms by avoiding spicy food, sugar, coffee, alcohol and fizzy drinks. Regular sleep and reducing stress can also help, as will eating fruit, vegetables and wholegrain cereals. Some people, however, find that too much cereal fibre, like bran, makes symptoms worse. Sufferers with excessive wind should also avoid too many beans and pulses. Natural yoghurt and probiotic yoghurt drinks can help, as they encourage 'good' gut bacteria. If these measures don't help, see your GP.

Heartburn, also called indigestion or acid reflux, is another common digestive problem. It happens when acid from the stomach comes back up the gullet. Lying down makes this more likely to happen, so symptoms are often worse at night. Apart from disturbing sleep patterns, acid reflux can inflame the lining of the food pipe in the throat. If you suffer from acid reflux, avoid eating a large meal close to bedtime. Cutting out alcohol and spicy food can also help. If these measures don't help, see your GP.

Inflammatory bowel disease or colitis can also be helped by eating regular small meals. Symptoms include frequent watery bowel movements that usually contain blood and mucus. Medical treatment is usually needed. Although what you eat will not cure the problem, it can affect the severity of symptoms. Make sure your diet is rich in anti-inflammatory nutrients, such as oily fish, green leafy vegetables, pumpkin seeds and pineapple.

'From a chiropractic perspective, there's often an important connection between spine alignment and digestion. Sorting out the back often helps the bowel.' **DR BEN**

Help! I'm flat-lining'

Has your weight loss slowed down or stopped? You're not alone – when weight has dropped off easily in the first few weeks, it's quite common for dieters to reach a bit of a plateau with no weight loss occurring for a while. We often see this happening around the 5–9 Week mark. So the first message is – don't worry!

'When I see someone who has reached a plateau, I ask them if they've inadvertently been eating more again, or if they've gone back to old patterns of skipping meals because they had too much to eat the day before, or if they've stopped fitting in as much exercise. I remind them to keep going with the plan, and usually the weight loss starts again after a week or two.' **PAM**

So the second message if you're flat-lining is to do something different. Look back at what you're eating and drinking. This will help you spot whether you've started getting a bit more generous with the portions. You might need to get the scales out and check that your estimation of 30g of cereal, for example, has not gradually approached 60g of cereal. If so, go back and read about portion distortion again (see pages 26–27).

You might also be slipping back into old habits, with the odd packet of crisps or bar of chocolate on the way home from work because you forgot to take a packet of raisins or a piece of fruit with you. Your dinner time might have slipped later and later, so that when you wake in the morning you're not hungry and skip breakfast. If so, make the effort to get back to three meals with two small, healthy snacks.

How are you getting on with your exercise? If it's been raining so you've not been for your walk, run or cycle ride, you might be flat-lining because you're using up less energy. There is a simple answer to this reason for flat-lining: get moving! Keep going and you'll soon see the weight drop off again.

'You can tackle flat-lining and kick-start renewed weight loss if you up the exercise.' **DR BEN**

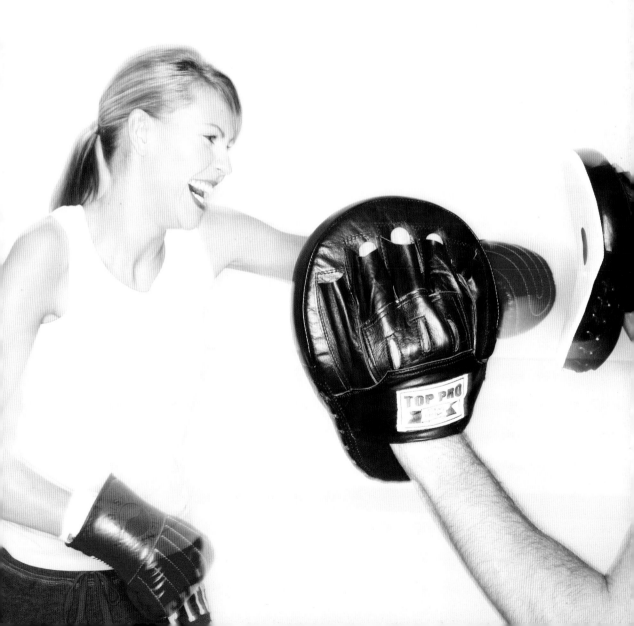

Shifting gear

As Dr Ben mentioned, a good trick for getting weight loss moving again when it has stalled for a while is to increase the intensity of the cardiovascular exercise you do. If you're walking for exercise, for example, that means you pick up the pace. If you were walking a mile in 25 minutes, speed up and try to complete it in 20 or 15 minutes. Or if you like cycling, go a bit faster or include a hill or two in your ride. Increasing the intensity of your exercise means you burn more calories during the exercise and the effect continues even when you've finished.

A good way to increase intensity is to use interval training. If you're doing a 30-minute walk, for example, walk at your normal pace for four and a half minutes, then run for 30 seconds. Repeat this pattern throughout the 30 minutes. This raises your heart rate but also stops you getting worn out too quickly. Gradually, you shift the balance so you run for a minute and walk for four minutes, working up to more time running than walking.

Another good way to increase intensity is to switch the activity to a more energetic one. So if you normally walk three times a week for your cardiovascular exercise, try replacing one or more session with swimming. Half an hour of brisk swimming takes a lot more energy than half an hour of brisk walking, which will help you shift the fat. Most pools also have kick boards and floats around – they let you swim using only your legs. Zooming up and down the pool visualizing your legs as an outboard motor will soon burn up the calories, as well as toning up the big leg muscles and the core muscles of the abdomen that give you a flat tum. If you feel a bit self-conscious going to a swimming pool, don't worry. Remember that it usually takes less than 30 seconds to get between the changing room and the pool, and nobody is there to judge you – they're at the pool for a workout, just like you.

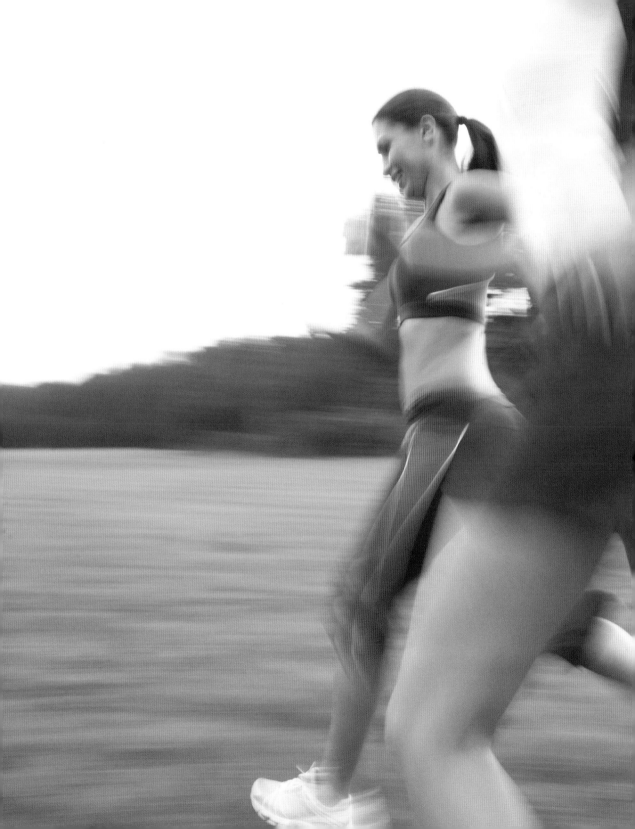

Week 5 6 7 8

Start the week

You're nearly two-thirds of the way through the 12-week diet plan. So check out your progress by weighing yourself. How does it compare with last week's weight? If you are following the rules and fitting in at least three sessions of exercise a week (as well as your daily range of stretching exercises) you should be losing about a pound a week. Look back at the rules on page 89 if you need a reminder.

Measurements chart

	LAST WEEK	NOW
Date	(__ /__ /__)	(__ /__ /__)
Weight		
Chest		
Waist		
Hips		
Others		
_____		
_____		
_____		

'I live with my husband and two teenage children, and what with seeing patients and looking after the family, like most working mothers I find time is short. But I always have breakfast as soon as I get up – eggs and mushrooms on wholegrain toast is one of my favourites, though sometimes there's only time for a bowl of cereal with fresh fruit, or a smoothie. After the morning rush and seeing a few patients, I usually have a mid-morning snack of a few nuts and an apple around 11 o'clock. I can't say I really love nuts, but they do make a handy snack as they're easy to carry around. I never eat at my computer or desk, so I tend to pop out for lunch in a café – something like a big bowl of green leafy salad with French beans, tomatoes, beetroot and anchovies. Sometimes, if I'm trying to fit in some shopping during my lunch hour, I grab a good quality sandwich. To keep me going until I get home, I have a natural yoghurt around 3.30 in the afternoon.

'I always cook a proper main meal every evening for the whole family. Family favourites include fish pie and spaghetti bolognaise. If I cook curry, it's usually vegetarian with lentils and spinach. I eat five portions of fruit and vegetables on most days. I have eggs at least two or three times a week, and a small amount of cheese. I have dessert occasionally, usually as part of Sunday lunch. We eat out quite often, but I don't usually eat the bread that is often brought at the beginning of the meal. I prefer to be hungry when my main meal comes so I can really enjoy it.

'I'm generally quite active, though I guess like a lot of mothers, much of the exercise I get seems to be when I'm doing jobs around the house: gardening, cleaning the house and tidying up. I walk from the surgery back to the station, and if it's a nice day, I get off a stop early to fit in an extra walk. I've been doing yoga for about 10 years. I'm a good swimmer, and fit in a trip to the pool most weeks. If the weather's good, I might go for a bike ride with my son, along the river. I walk quite a lot, but I've never mastered the art of running – I can run quite fast for 200 yards but 400 yards is probably the furthest I can manage without collapsing!'

'Help! I'm bored with it all'

It's nearly two months since you started the 12-week diet plan, so the novelty might be wearing off. But that's not a reason to give up – it's a signal that you are ready to move on to something new. You might be ready to start the next phase of the diet plan and the exercise programme – if so, skip ahead and see what's in store. Then get started! Not a problem. Your body is probably ready for the next challenge.

Are you a bit bored with the food you're eating? Again, if you need some new ideas of what to eat, take a peep at page 128 where we show you the next part of the plan. The healthy eating principles still apply, but we've made some different recipe suggestions to give your taste buds some new sensations. So cook a meal you've never cooked before. There is a huge range of colourful fruit and vegetables just waiting to be tried – you don't know which ones you will love until you taste them. Spend some time browsing round the stalls in a street market, or checking out the vegetable aisles in the supermarket and buy something that takes your fancy. You'll soon stop feeling bored if you try something different.

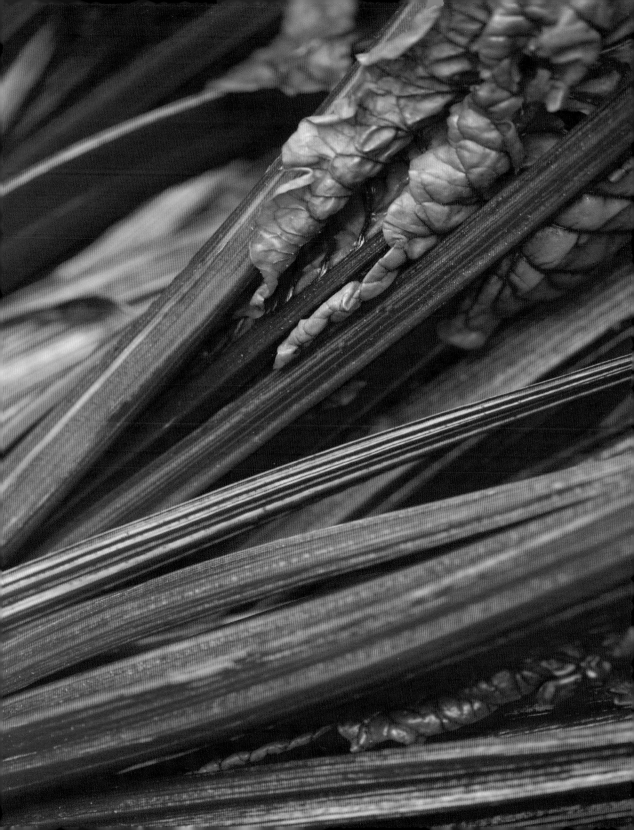

Allergy alert

The increase in allergic diseases is often in the news, with reports of more people than ever before suffering from allergic asthma (allergy affecting the lungs), eczema (allergy affecting the skin) and hayfever (allergy affecting the nose and sinuses). Allergies occur when the body's immune system over-reacts to something in the environment – usually things like house dust mites, pet hair or grass pollen. But food allergy is probably the biggest worry. Each year, around 3000 people in the UK are admitted to hospital with severe allergies to food, and sadly it proves fatal in around 20 people each year.

Finding out what causes the allergy requires careful detective work, using food diaries to record everything that is eaten and drunk, and blood tests to check reactions to possible causes, so the culprit can be identified. Although many tests are available from various organizations, they're not always very reliable, so it is better to discuss any possible food allergies with your GP.

Common trigger foods are peanuts, other nuts like almonds and walnuts, and shellfish. Using a food diary showed that one of the recent contributors to *The Diet Doctors: Inside and Out* had a reaction to diet cola that caused her lips and face to swell. It was most likely an additive or preservative that caused the problem. Anyone with a food allergy needs to avoid the trigger food, so we advised her to stay off the fizz!

In someone with a food allergy, eating the trigger food (or drink), or sometimes even just touching it, can cause an immediate reaction with an itchy rash, swelling of the mouth and face, breathing difficulties and collapse. Emergency treatment is needed if this occurs, and an ambulance should be called immediately. Anyone who has suffered a bad allergic reaction to food should carry an adrenaline injector pen for emergency use, and family, friends and colleagues should know how to administer it too, in case the sufferer collapses and is unable to use it themselves.

Fortunately, most bad reactions to food are not allergies; they're due to food intolerance. These reactions occur hours or days after eating the trigger food, and are not life-threatening. Food intolerance commonly causes diarrhoea, vomiting, bloating, flatulence and headaches, but can also cause other symptoms. Intolerance to wheat and some other cereals that contain gluten is known as coeliac disease. Another common cause of intolerance is to the lactose in dairy products. Finding out what causes intolerance is even more difficult than identifying the cause of a food allergy. Although the culprit should be removed from the diet, it is important to ensure that essential nutrients are not excluded, so consult your GP for help, if you suspect you are intolerant to a certain food.

If you think you often suffer from diarrhoea, bloating, headaches and just generally feeling horrible, and you think it might be due to what you are eating, it's worth seeing the impact of our 12-week diet plan. We often find that eating regular, healthy meals with small snacks in between sorts out this vague not-well feeling. Cutting out ready-made meals, processed foods and snacks with no nutritional value, and replacing them with freshly prepared foods packed with vitamins and minerals can quickly restore a real sense of wellbeing – look back at page 74 if you need a reminder on why they matter. Getting into good eating habits can also help, as we discussed on page 73, so that delicate stomachs are not alternately stuffed and starved!

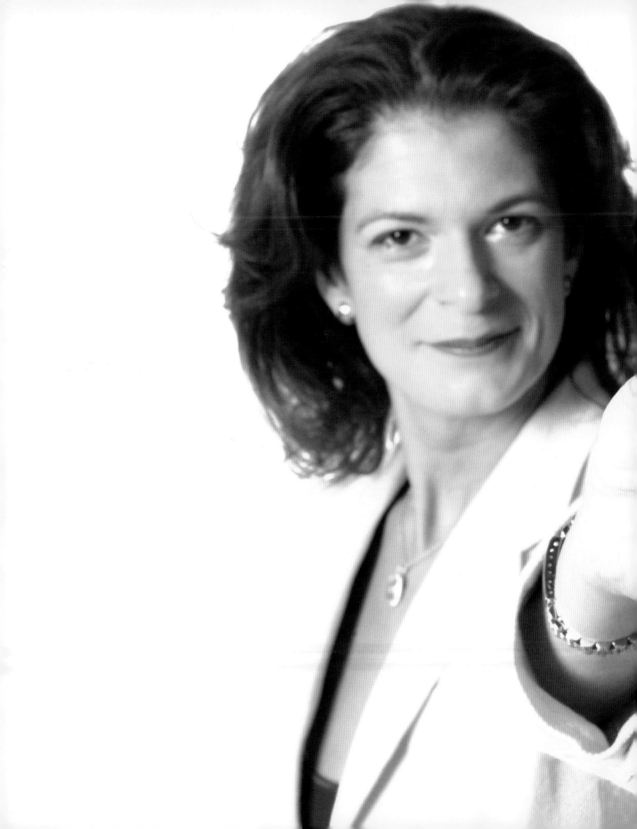

CHAPTER 5

Weeks
9–12

What's going to happen this month?

You've now reached the final stage of the 12-week diet plan. During the first few weeks you concentrated on changing basic habits, and settling into a regular pattern of eating three healthy and well-balanced meals each day, with a couple of nutritious mini-snacks to make sure you don't get too hungry. So you should find that there's now no need to reach for crisps, chocolates or biscuits. During the last month, you will have broadened the range of foods that you eat. With all the vitamins and minerals in your diet, you should be feeling energetic and have a greater sense of well being.

So now it's time to move into the third phase of the 12-week diet plan. You will be continuing with all the changes you have already made to your diet, but we also want you to increase the number of non-meat meals that you eat. This is to help reduce the amount of saturated fats you are eating, as these are mainly found in meat and other animal products.

We've included a number of vegetarian meal suggestions for you to try. In vegetarian meals, the protein required is often provided by nuts and seeds. These ingredients also boost the amount of essential omega unsaturated oils that you eat, helping your blood vessels to stay healthy.

This month, we also want you to tone up your body more. Your body should now be more flexible and able to cope with strengthening exercises. These exercises will also make sure that the weight you lose comes from fat and not from muscle. They will help you shape up and look good.

During this final month, you should lose another 4lbs. At the end of week 12, you will be able to see your progress when you weigh yourself again, take your measurements and repeat the flexibility assessment. As before, you will be able to record your progress.

The rules for weeks 9–12

1. Eat three meals and two healthy snacks every day. Remember to include a little protein each time

2. Eat five portions of fruit and vegetables every day

3. Eat at least two portions of fish a week

4. Eat more non-meat meals

5. Eat no more than one portion of high fat, high sugar food a week

6. Always keep an eye on your portion sizes

7. Keep drinking water

8. Continue to limit your alcohol intake

9. Do your Daily Stretching Routine on pages 60–61

10. Aim to walk 10,000 steps a day

11. Exercise your heart and lungs at least three times every week

12. Tone up your body with strengthening exercises at least three times a week

13. Weigh and measure yourself once a week only

14. Keep up your food and mood diary

Week 9 10 11 12

Start the week

You've now completed 2 months of the 12-week diet plan and it's time to see how much progress you have made since you started the plan. Fill in your original weight and measurements then step on the scales and get out your tape measure to record your current weight and measurements. Are you pleased with the difference? You should be making steady progress towards your goal, with a total weight loss of 8lbs or more.

Now repeat the flexibility test on pages 30–31. After another month of daily your range of stretching exercises, you should notice further improvement in your score. You will also feel fitter, after 8 weeks of walking more and 4 weeks of regular cardiovascular exercise. If you've been sticking to the rules you should really be noticing the benefits on your weight, health and wellbeing.

If you haven't managed to lose at least half a stone, think back over the last month and try to work out why. Have you slipped back to old habits? Have your portion sizes crept back up? Have you missed too many exercise sessions? It is never too late to start following the plan, so look back at the rules for this month, and take the steps required to shape up for the future. You know you'll look slimmer, be healthier and feel great if you follow the 12-week diet plan.

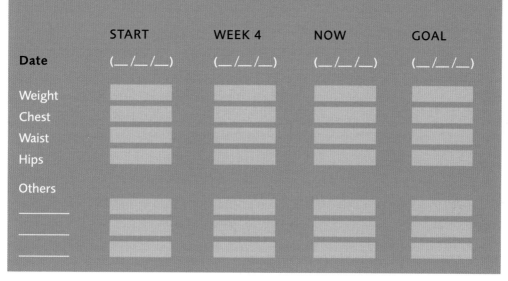

Measurements chart

	START (__ / __ / __)	WEEK 4 (__ / __ / __)	NOW (__ / __ / __)	GOAL (__ / __ / __)
Date				
Weight				
Chest				
Waist				
Hips				
Others				
_____				
_____				
_____				

What's on the menu?

Although you need to eat some meat each week to ensure a healthy intake of essential nutrients, the fat in meat can be turned into unhealthy cholesterol that can damage your blood vessels (see page 105). You may already be eating less meat because you have increased the amount of fish you are eating. But you may want to have a vegetarian meal once or twice a week. Well-balanced vegetarian meals should include beans, pulses (like lentils), nuts, cheese or dairy products like milk or yoghurt. Many vegetarian meals are quick and easy to make, and there's plenty of scope for lots of flavour. You will still need to take care that you don't eat too large a portion of rice or pasta, but portions can be a little larger than for rice or pasta dishes that include fish or meat.

VEGETARIAN SUGGESTIONS
(see recipes starting on page 192)

RICE AND PASTA DISHES

Green risotto with runner beans, peas and spinach

Linguine with sweet potato, feta cheese and rocket

Pasta with aubergines and peppers

SALADS AND OTHER IDEAS

ABC salad

Green bean and pimiento salad

Seasonal roasted vegetables with yoghurt couscous

Arabic feast

Baked sweet potato

CURRIES AND SPICY DISHES

Lentil curry in a hurry

DESSERT SUGGESTIONS
(see recipes starting on page 202)

Fresh fruit salad

Grilled mango

Strawberries dipped in chocolate

Cinnamon baked apple with cranberries

Since you started the diet plan, you should have ditched the cakes, biscuits, sweets, ice creams and other puddings and desserts, in favour of fruit or yoghurt. But if you are desperate for a dessert, there are many fruit-based dishes that won't blow the diet. We've given you some suggestions here, but look through some cook books for other ideas. Just make sure that you give those based on cream and sugar a miss.

Keep moving

You've now reached the third phase of the exercise plan. You should already notice an improvement in your health and fitness thanks to your daily walking and stretching routines and the additional cardio workouts you are doing three times a week. This month we are adding to the basic mix of range of movement and cardiovascular exercises by introducing strengthening exercises to tone your body. As with any kind of exercise, if you have any concerns, check with your doctor or chiropractor.

You can do simple exercises at home to strengthen all your muscles, without needing special equipment or too much time – just 10–30 minutes will be sufficient to tone you up. You might want to do the strengthening exercises given below, after you've done the range of movement exercises that you started in the first month. Or you might prefer a different time of the day. It's up to you. Just try and make sure that you do strengthening exercises at least three times a week.

When you are doing the strengthening exercises, if you've not just done the stretching exercises, then warm up first by gently swinging your arms and walking on the spot. Wear comfortable clothing and make sure you have carpeted floor to lie on, or a rug or exercise mat – we don't want you to be uncomfortable. Keep breathing slowly and steadily throughout. Take it easy, particularly during the first week, and gradually build up.

1. LUNGE

Stand upright with your feet shoulder width apart and place your hands on your hips. Pull in your tummy. Take a long step forwards, landing on the ball of your foot, and bend your front knee. Keep your body upright and make sure you don't drop your head or shoulders forwards. Pause and then return to the starting position by stepping back with the front leg. Repeat with the other leg. Start with just a few lunges on each side, and gradually increase until you are able to do 10–15 on each leg.

2. SQUATS

Stand upright with your feet shoulder width apart. Pull in your tummy. Bending your legs, slowly lower your backside as if you were going to sit on a chair. Keep your weight directly over your heels and raise your arms to shoulder height to give you balance. Go as low as you feel able, but make sure your backside always remains higher than your knees. Pause, then slowly return to the starting position. Repeat, starting with just a few, and gradually increase until you are able to do 20–30.

3. CRUNCHES

Now lie down on your back on the floor with your knees bent and your feet flat on the floor hip width apart. Put your thumbs on the bottom of your ribcage and your index fingers on the points at the front of your pelvis. Slowly curl up and try to lift your head, neck and shoulder blades off the floor, without causing strain to your neck. Pull in your tummy by bringing your thumb and index fingers close together. Remember, it's not how high you get your shoulders off the floor – we want the abdominal muscles across the front of your tummy to do the work! Pause, and then slowly return to the starting position. Repeat, starting with just a few, and gradually increase until you are able to do 20–30.

4. BACK EXTENSION

Roll over so that you are face down. Put your arms down by your sides with the palms facing up, and have your legs extended and relaxed. Relax your shoulders into the floor. Pull in your tummy – imagine that there's a strawberry under your belly button that you don't want to squash! Now squeeze your buttocks together and slowly lift your shoulders and chest off the floor. Let your head come up too but keep your eyes facing forwards so you don't arch your neck. Pause, then slowly return to the starting position. Repeat, starting with just a few, and gradually increase until you are able to do up to 12. To rest your back after this exercise, you might want to take your backside back over your toes, bending your knees so that your body lies face down, your back is nicely rounded and your arms lie straight in front of you.

5. PLANK

Lying face down with your legs stretched out, bend your arms so that your elbows are next to your body and your hands, palms down, are next to your shoulders. Curl your toes under and pull in your tummy. Now push up keeping your forearms on the floor, so that your body weight is supported on your toes and lower arms. Keep your body straight – like a plank – without pushing your backside into the air. Hold the position for just a few seconds to begin with, but over time you might manage to hold for 30–60 seconds. Slowly lower your body to the floor.

6. PUSH-UPS

Don't let push-ups frighten you! You can start with an easy version then work your way up to doing full push-ups. Begin with standing 2 feet away from a table or kitchen bench, and place your hands securely on the edge of the table or bench, shoulder width apart. Bend your elbows and lower your chest between your hands towards the table or bench and then push back up to straighten your arms. Aim to do 10, building up to 25.

If you find these easy to do, progress to knee push-ups. Lie face down on the floor, with hands beside your shoulders. Push up to straighten your arms whilst keeping your knees on the ground. Aim to do 10, building up to 25. When you have the strength, try a full push-up by using the same technique as a knee push-up but straighten your legs so that when you use your arms to push up, your whole body is off the ground and your weight is supported by your hands and the balls of your feet. Aim to do 10, building up to 25.

7. BALANCE AND STRETCH

Kneel on all fours with your hands beneath your shoulders, your knees directly under your hips and your back flat. Pull in your tummy. Without lifting your head, slowly lift one arm in front of you while stretching out and lifting the opposite leg behind you. Make sure that you do not roll to one side. Pause, then slowly return to the starting position and repeat with the other arm and leg. Repeat, starting with just a few and gradually increase until you are able to do up to 10 on each side.

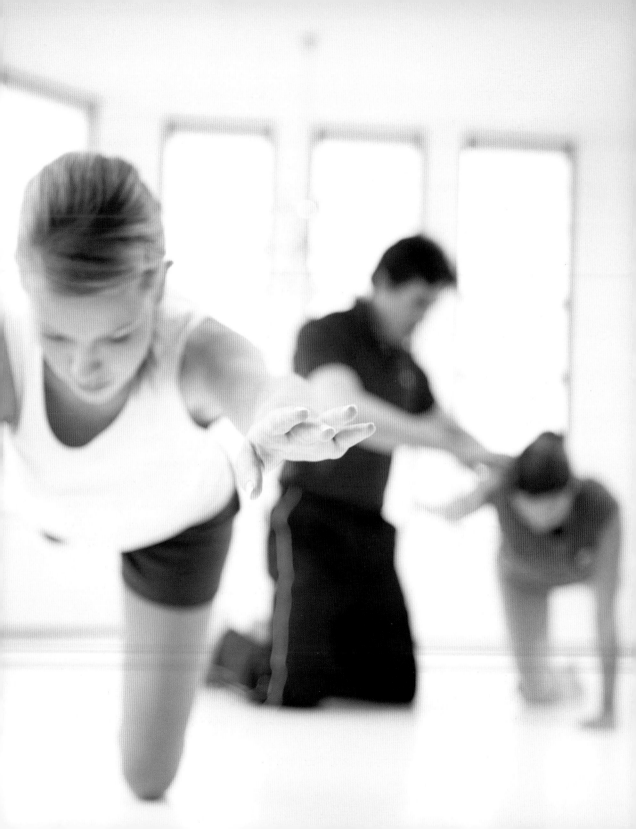

8. CAT STRETCH

Now a nice easy one to finish off with and give you a bit of a rest, while gently working your back. This is an excellent exercise if you have any back problems. Kneel on all fours, with your hands directly beneath your shoulders and your knees directly under your hips. With a flat back, pull in your tummy. Slowly drop your head between your arms and round your back to form a 'C' shape. Now, still with your tummy pulled in and without pausing, return to a flat back and then lift your head upwards, and push your backside upwards too, so that your back curves the opposite way. Without pausing, move slowly back to the flat back position and then the 'C' shape. Continue for up to 10 cycles.

As you gain confidence, you might want to do other forms of strengthening exercises, replacing one or more of your at-home sessions so that you maintain at least three sessions a week. You could join a yoga or Pilates class – the exercises here are based on Pilates which is a gentle way to strengthen and tone your body. Just look in your local paper to find a suitable class. You might also want to join a gym where you can use resistance machines or free weights to increase muscle strength and tone. Make sure, though, that you are shown what to do by an instructor so that you know how to exercise without causing yourself any harm.

THOUGHT FOR THE WEEK

'If you're overweight, your body is under a huge strain. It means it's going to wear out an awful lot quicker. Shed the extra pounds and take away that strain on your body. You'll feel so much better.' DR BEN

'Help! I'm going on holiday'

If you don't want to see the pounds piling back on, it makes sense to plan ahead before you go. Let's start with food. It's always tempting to splurge on holiday, but try to stick to the same pattern of eating when you're away. It's easier to eat healthily on holiday than you think, and remember that if you really fancy indulging, you can always share your portion to keep the calories down!

If you're going on a self-catering holiday, potter round local markets and choose colourful fruit and vegetables to try. Make it part of the holiday to experiment. If you're staying in a hotel, most now include breakfast buffets, so you can choose from an array of cereals, dried fruits and other healthy goodies – you don't have to go for fried egg, bacon and sausage just because they are on offer. If you enjoy a big cooked breakfast, that's not a problem – we want you to have breakfast. Just choose boiled or scrambled egg rather than fried, and have the mushrooms and tomatoes rather than the hash browns and sausages.

When it comes to eating out in the evening, choose carefully so you can enjoy your meal without overdoing it. Make the most of fish and shellfish. Salad and grilled meat like steak or chicken breast are also safe options and in line with the plan – but keep an eye on portions and be prepared to leave some if the helping is too large. And remember, you don't have to have an ice cream every day – once a week can feel like enough of a treat.

When it comes to exercise, you can still do your flexibility and strength exercises, as they don't need any equipment. Many holiday resorts and hotels include great gym facilities, and swimming in a pool or sea can be refreshing as well as good exercise. You could even try out new sports or activities – horse riding on the beach? Windsurfing? Waterskiing? Whatever you do make sure you enjoy it!

Week 9 10 11 12

Start the week

There's just a few weeks left before you reach the end of the 12-week diet plan, so hop on the scales to see how you are getting on then get out your tape measure to record your body measurements. Fill in your details in the chart below.

Read the rules for the month again, to make sure that you know what you are doing. Notice the rule about drinking. Are you managing this? We'll be looking at the calories in drink this week.

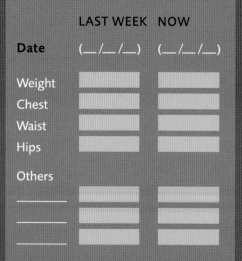

Measurements chart

	LAST WEEK	NOW
Date	(__ /__ /__)	(__ /__ /__)
Weight		
Chest		
Waist		
Hips		
Others		
_____		
_____		
_____		

Drink up

What you drink, whether it's alcoholic or non-alcoholic, can affect your ability to lose weight. You can see what we mean if your day goes anything like this:

- Start the day with a refreshing orange juice (58 calories) and a probiotic shot to feed up the good gut bacteria (75 calories).
- Grab a tall cappuccino on the way to work (150 calories).
- Feel virtuous about getting one of your 'five a day' in a mid-morning fruit smoothie (190 calories).
- Break for lunch, which includes a can of fizzy drink (139 calories).
- Meet up with a friend on the way home for work, having a hot chocolate (330 calories).
- Arrive home, sip a refreshing glass of cranberry juice while you make the dinner (140 calories)
- Enjoy a medium glass of white wine with dinner (132 calories).
- Round off the day with a nice warming malty bedtime drink made with semi-skimmed milk (211 calories).

All seems pretty reasonable, don't you think? Well, yes, but the liquid calories add up to nearly 1500 – that's three-quarters of the average woman's daily limit of 2000 and more than half the average man's daily requirement of 2500 calories. Now that wouldn't result in a weight problem if the average woman, drinking all of the drinks listed above, ate only a bowl of cereal and a sandwich – though she might be compromising her health due to lack of vitamins. But the reality is, as we all know, that she's likely to be eating a full range of meals, and quite possibly muffins alongside the hot chocolate! So what happens to all the extra calories she's consuming? They piles on as pounds. She tells her friends that she can't understand why she's putting on weight as she's not eating very much – and she's right, the extra calories are in what she's drinking.

So if you're finding weight difficult to shift, think back to what you're drinking. Can you replace any drinks that are giving you little nutritional benefit (such as the fizzy drink, cappuccino or hot chocolate) with refreshing sparkling water or herbal tea that don't add to your calories? Remember that a spoon of sugar in every cup of tea, quite apart from damaging your teeth soon mounts up to a lot of calories.

And while we are on the subject of drinks, let's spend a few minutes on alcohol. A small amount of red wine a week is probably good for your heart, as well as being enjoyable, though drinking alcohol has been linked with an increase in some cancers. But there are a number of other problems with drinking alcohol when you want to lose weight. For a start, there are the calories packed into each glass which can quickly blow your energy budget sky-high. Then there's the problem of how one glass can lead to another and the next thing you know, you've drunk the whole bottle, multiplying the calorie problem. And then there is the problem of what you choose to eat when you drink – who says 'no' to the crisps or peanuts passed around, or 'no' to stopping off for a curry on the way home, when they're worse for wear? The next day, a hangover

can play havoc with sensible eating as so your regular eating patterns can get all distorted.

If you are struggling to shift those pounds, it's better to lay off the booze, at least until you've reached your target weight. You might also want to think about the impact of regular drinking on your health. Alcohol is a poison which has to be detoxified by the liver. Drinking steadily every day, or binge drinking large amounts, can exhaust your liver, so that it gets damaged and cirrhosis sets in. The first signs may be hard to spot – a vague feeling of being tired and unwell, nausea, swollen ankles, yellowish tinge to the eyes – though your doctor may detect it using a blood test. To reduce the risk of liver damage, women should drink no more than 14 units of alcohol per week – that's no more than one small (125ml) glass of wine a day. Men should drink no more than 21 units of alcohol per week – that's less than a pint of strong beer a night. But remember these are maximum amounts, not levels to be aimed for. The less alcohol you drink, the less risk of certain cancers.

Get the measure of alcoholic drinks

DRINKS	APPROXIMATE CALORIES	APPROXIMATE UNITS
White wine		
Small glass (125ml)	94	1.6
Medium glass (175ml)	132	2.2
Large glass (250ml)	188	3.25
Red wine		
Small glass (125ml)	85	1.6
Medium glass (175ml)	119	2.2
Large glass (250ml)	170	3.25
Beer and lager		
Half a pint standard lager (4%)	83	1.1
Half a pint strong lager (5%)	83	1.4
Pint draught bitter	184	2
Spirits		
Gin (23ml) and tonic (110ml)	85	1
Vodka (40%)	53	1
Alcopops	160–220	1.5

You can calculate the number of units in any alcoholic drink by multiplying the percentage alcohol (always given on the label) by the volume of drink in ml, and dividing by 1000.

'Help! I'm going to a party'

Everyone enjoys going to a party, but it's a good idea to think ahead so you can plan how to have a good time without piling the pounds back on.

Before you go to the party, make sure you have eaten something. We know the temptation might be to 'save up' for the food and booze by skimping yourself during the day, but it just doesn't work. If you arrive at the party with an empty stomach, that first glass of something will go straight to your head and knock out all thoughts about being careful. And you'll also be unable to resist the canapés or nibbles. Far better to have a small protein-based meal that will stay in your stomach for some time, such as a boiled egg with granary bread toast or a baked potato with tuna and mayonnaise. This will slow the absorption of alcohol and stop hunger pangs from getting out of control. Try to alternate alcoholic drinks with water, to keep the calories down and prevent you losing control of what you are doing. Have fun!

Ironing out problems

We see many women who are run down and tired all the time because they are short of iron. This is needed in red blood cells to transport oxygen around the blood, and for other important processes in the body. Without iron, every day feels like scaling Everest without an air supply.

If you're tired and lacking energy, check you aren't suffering from iron shortage – your doctor can arrange a simple blood test. Although there are many other reasons for problems with red blood cells most common cause of anaemia is iron deficiency. Your GP can prescribe iron supplements. Some types can lead to constipation, but other types in liquid form cause fewer problems.

A good diet can help you get enough iron. Increase the amount of red meat you eat, such as beef and lamb, as these contain a lot of iron that is easy to absorb. Liver is also an extremely good source, though it should be eaten in moderation as with turkey and shellfish. However, don't eat liver or raw shellfish if you are pregnant.

You can also get iron from some fruit and vegetables, though this is harder to absorb than iron from meat or shellfish. Broccoli, kale, parsley, watercress and other dark green leafy vegetables contain iron, as do dried fruits such as raisins, figs, prunes and dates. Baked beans, and other types of cooked beans and lentils, have reasonably high levels of iron.

Eating fruit and vegetable sources in the same meal as red meat increases the amount of iron your body can extract from food. You'll also absorb more if you start meals with orange or tomato juice, grapefruit or melon, and finish off with strawberries or an orange. On the other hand, drinking red wine with meals reduces the amount of iron your body absorbs. Tea, coffee and drinks containing caffeine like cola also reduce absorption.

THOUGHT FOR THE WEEK

'A good diet can't cure every illness, but it can prevent a lot of them.' PAM

Week 9 10 **11** 12

Start the week

You're almost there! Start the week well by recording your weight and measurements in the box below. If you need to, look back at the rules for the month (page 125). You should be aiming to lose another pound this week.

Measurements chart

	LAST WEEK	NOW
Date	(__ /__ /__)	(__ /__ /__)
Weight		
Chest		
Waist		
Hips		
Others		
_____		
_____		
_____		

Mood food

Did you know that scientific studies have proved food affects mood? Eating well has been shown to reduce depression, mood swings, anxiety and panic attacks. After 11 weeks on the diet plan, you may have already noticed this yourself. We also regularly hear that our diet plan improves mood, and one of the contributors to *The Diet Doctors: Inside and Out* was able to come off antidepressants after a month of eating regularly and well, as she no longer needed them. However, it's important to mention that you should never change your dose of anti-depressants without consulting your doctor, even if you feel your mood improving.

Protein, complex carbohydrates and the omega fats alongside vitamins and minerals such as vitamin C, folic acid, vitamin B6, B12, and zinc are needed for good mental health. They are found individually in a variety of foods such as watercress, avocado, nuts and seeds, dried apricot and oily fish. Refined sugars can raise your blood glucose too quickly, leading to a slump later on, which in some people has been shown to lead to mood changes and symptoms such as anxiety and irritability.

Regular exercise, particularly outdoors, can also help increase a general sense of wellbeing. It leads to the production of feel-good chemicals in the brain. So as you power walk across the park, remember it's not just your body you're helping, but your soul as well.

'I'm not perfect with my health all the time, but I do stick to the 80/20 rule – I keep on track 80 per cent of the time.' DR BEN

On the bread line

Over the last few years, high-protein/ low-carbohydrate diets have been popular, taking bread off the menu for many people. However, the good news is that bread is back. While we don't think it's a good idea to have too much bread if you want to lose weight, a couple of slices a day is a good way of getting vital vitamins.

There is some great bread in the shops nowadays, but you need to choose carefully. Try to avoid processed white sliced bread. The refining process used to make white flour takes away most of the nutrients. The bread manufacturers are legally obliged to add extra vitamins and minerals, to make up for what has been taken away, but it's better to eat wholemeal bread made with the complete wheat grain, which contains more iron and three times more zinc than white bread. Wholegrain bread also contains more fibre, so that eating it leaves you feeling fuller for longer than white bread. So use your loaf when it comes to bread.

'Help! I've had a blow-out and put the weight back on'

It can happen! But, before you overreact and turn back to comfort eating big time, stop and think. One big night out might mean that you've put back a couple of pounds, but that's not a disaster. One bad day won't undermine all the health benefits of eating food with more vitamins and minerals during the last few weeks. You are probably following our 12-week diet plan not just because of your weight, but also because of your health. One overeating session won't make much difference to your overall wellbeing.

So now you've got it into perspective, what are you going to do? You could use the overeating as an excuse to go back to your old ways, so that you *definitely* put weight back on. Or you could accept that it happened, put it behind you, and get back to eating sensibly and healthily. Then any weight you've put back on because of your blow-out will be removed again. And you could also try to look at the reasons for why it happened, so that you can guard against another bout of overeating. Whatever you do, don't skip your meals the next day.

Hormones and health

Hormones regulate many processes in the body, and when they get out of balance, a whole host of problems can set in.

If you're struggling to lose weight despite following the diet plan (without cheating!), you may have a problem with your thyroid gland. If this is underactive, you may feel cold and tired all the time, and have general hair loss, dry skin and constipation. Your thyroid needs iodine to function properly, which can be found in seafood and garlic. Selenium is another important mineral, found in nuts (particularly brazil and cashew nuts), cooked fish, lentils, hummus, mushrooms and seeds (such as sesame and sunflower). Foods rich in zinc can also help – so up the amount of almonds, pumpkin seeds, chicken, turkey, crab and oysters in your diet. If you are concerned, consult your doctor.

Another common hormonal problem in overweight women is polycystic ovary syndrome (PCOS). In PCOS, the male and female sex hormones get out of balance. Cysts can develop in the ovaries and ovulation can be erratic, so women with this condition may have difficulty getting pregnant. Other signs of PCOS include excessive facial hair, acne and irregular periods. Women with PCOS tend to store fat around their waist, and this is often linked to problems with the hormone insulin, which can result in diabetes (see page 82). Although PCOS makes it difficult to lose weight, shifting the extra pounds is thought to alleviate some of the symptoms and help reduce the risk of developing diabetes.

If you think you might have PCOS, see your GP and eat three meals and two healthy snacks everyday to keep blood sugar levels as steady as possible. Eat more foods rich in chromium (egg yolks, wholegrains, seeds, liver and kidney) and zinc (shellfish, chickpeas, oats and sardines), both of which are important.

HOW DOES DR BEN DO IT?

'I don't really have a typical day – some days I see patients but other days I'm with the Leicester Tigers or England rugby teams. On a day I'm in the clinic, I usually wake up around 6 o'clock and do some stretches. I then drink half a litre of warm water, sometimes with freshly squeezed lemon juice. This wakes up my digestion and gets me rehydrated.

'After a shower, I do the flexibility exercises on pages 60–61. By 6.30 I'm having breakfast. This might be porridge or a couple of slices of granary toast with olive oil (rather than butter), topped with tomato and smoked salmon or a poached egg.

'I'm out the door by 7 o'clock and seeing patients by 8 o'clock. Adjusting spines and limbs is quite physical work, so during the morning I'll usually drink about 600ml of water, sometimes with lemon, and a cup of green tea. By 10 o'clock I'm ravenous, so I usually have a toasted panini. I pop out to a deli to get my snack, so I also get a breath of air. I have a lunch break at 1 o'clock.

Sometimes I fetch a salad or a salmon or egg sandwich. In the afternoon, I see patients. I drink another 600ml of water, and sometimes green tea. I'll often have a piece of fruit or a handful of seeds and nuts. I usually leave by 7pm, and I'm home by 7.30.

'Dinner is often a combination of things prepared at the weekend, or I fix an Arabic feast or green curry. I eat a lot of organic salmon, sardines and other fish. I was a vegetarian for eight years, but now I eat meat occasionally when I'm out, mainly game or beef – I just felt that I needed more protein.

'I believe it's imperative to make exercise a priority so I aim to fit in at least three 30-minute sessions a week. For me, exercise is not a chore, as I only do what I enjoy. I don't like pumping iron in a gym, but I belong to a boxing gym and go there a couple of times a week. I also fence, and play rugby socially. I might go to a yoga or Pilates class or salsa dancing, or for a walk in the park at the weekend.'

Week 9 10 11 12

Start the week

You're starting the last week of the 12-week diet plan now, so it's a good time to check out your progress. Weigh yourself and record the details. Remind yourself of the rules on page 125, and try to lose one more pound this week. At the end of the week, you'll be able to take your measurements and repeat the flexibility test to see just how far you have come during the 12-week diet plan.

Measurements chart

	LAST WEEK	NOW
Date	(__/__/__)	(__/__/__)
Weight		
Chest		
Waist		
Hips		
Others		
_____		
_____		
_____		

Dear diary ...

You've reached the last week of the 12-week diet plan. You should have turned around your eating and exercising habits, improved your health and fitness, and lost some weight. So you can see just what's changed, we would like you to keep a food diary again this week, just as you did at the beginning of the 12-week period. Then you will be able to compare the two, and see just how far you've come. So get out your notebook, and start recording everything that you eat and drink, the time and the place, and how you felt. At the end of the week, score yourself again, using the healthy eating questionnaire on page 35.

Bend and stretch

If you have any form of arthritis, you will know that inflammation in the joints can make them stiff and painful. Understandably, this can make you reluctant to move the joint, to minimize the pain. However, lack of movement itself can lead to further stiffness. So gentle mobility exercises, carried out each day, are very important to maintain and extend the range of movement, and improve the health of the joints. The exercises started in the first week of the 12-week diet plan should be suitable for most people with arthritis, though it makes sense to check first with a chiropractor or doctor. Exercising in water is particularly helpful, as the joints are supported.

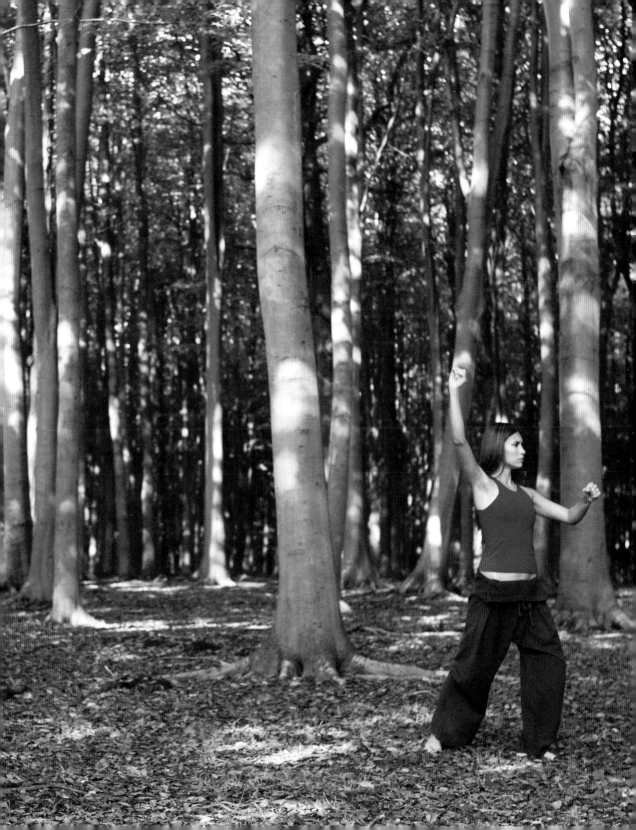

'Help! It's Christmas'

If it's getting all the shopping done, we know why you're concerned! But we suspect you're worried you'll blow all the success of the last few weeks.

It's important to remember that Christmas (or other important festivals that involve lots of eating, like Diwali and Hanukkah) come only once each year! It's what you do over the rest of the year that matters most. Having said that, Christmas now seems to be stretching from the end of November to the middle of January. It's one thing to overeat on Christmas Day and Boxing Day, but quite another if you overeat from November to January. If you are going to eat and drink too much, make sure you restrict it to only a few days.

A big problem with Christmas, or the other big festive occasions, is all that temptation. Christmas lunch is actually a very nutritious meal, with a great array of vegetables. So it's not a problem if your plate is piled high with Brussels sprouts and carrots – it's only a problem if it's sky high with roast potatoes and bread sauce. The real difficulty lies in the chocolates, the mince pies and the fridge bursting with all those tasty morsels. Even though it's Christmas, stick to eating three meals each day with fruit and vegetables covering around half of the plate, and your meat or fish and potatoes or rice covering the other half (in a single layer!). Eat the goodies as part of your meals or snacks. Try to limit puds and sweets to a few mouthfuls – and you don't have to take a chocolate every time the tin is passed round. Remember that if you overindulge, you need to get out and burn off those extra chocolates. A brisk walk is a great way to use up the extra energy – it will make you feel much better than sitting on the sofa in front of an old film, groaning from an over-full stomach.

The other big problem with Christmas is drink. Try to stick to just one alcoholic drink at each party or celebratory meal. Keep a glass in your hand so you've got something to sip, but make sure it's sparkling water or a fruity cocktail. Then you'll keep a clear head so you can really enjoy the festive period and emerge in January still able to fit into your party clothes and feeling healthy.

Damping the fire

Surprising as it may seem, rheumatoid arthritis that makes joints stiff and swollen, itchy skin conditions such as dermatitis, and the breathing problem, asthma, all have something in common. They can all be the result of inflammatory reactions in the body, with the immune system triggered to react inappropriately. If you suffer from an inflammatory condition, you may need medication from your doctor to control your symptoms. But simple changes to your diet can help as well.

You are probably already doing this, but try to reduce the amount of saturated fats in your diet by cutting back on the amount of red meat, takeaways and ready meals that you eat. It can help to cut back on coffee and other drinks that contain caffeine such as cola – switch to green tea. While it's a good idea to limit alcoholic drinks, a small glass of red wine each day may be beneficial for some people, so monitor the effect of alcohol on your symptoms. Go steady on spicy and sugary foods as these may aggravate inflammatory conditions.

Make sure that the food you eat includes lots of the right kind of fats, found in salmon, sea bass, mackerel, sardines and flax seeds. Choose olive oil to cook with, rather than lard or butter. Boost your vitamin C intake by eating lots of fruit and vegetables, but it might be better to avoid citrus fruits. Vitamin E is also important, found in seeds, nuts, eggs and brown rice. Try to include ginger, garlic, onions, asparagus and pineapple in your diet as these all contain natural anti-inflammatory compounds.

How have you got on?

Congratulations! You've now completed the 12-week diet plan. If you've stuck to the 12-week diet plan, you should have lost around a stone in weight. You will be looking slimmer. You will have significantly improved your health. Most important of all, you will be feeling better.

There's no doubt about it, if you've lost weight in the healthy way we've shown you in the 12-week diet plan, you'll have improved your body on the inside and outside.

It's time to take a look at just how far you have come. Fill in your original weight and measurements in the table below then step on the scales and get out the tape measure. How close are you to your goal weight? Have you got much further to go? Take another picture of yourself and compare it to the one you took at the beginning. Are you pleased with the difference?

Go back to page 35 and take the Healthy Eating Test again. You should score much higher this time round. This is because you have increased the amount of healthy and nutritious food you are eating and slashed the food stacked high with calories but lacking nutrients. These changes will have improved your health, regardless of your weight. (And your fridge will have had a makeover too!)

Now try out the flexibility test again. Do you see a difference? Compare your score to the one when you first took the test. If you have exercised regularly, you should have noticed a real increase in your body's range of movement. All the walking and the exercises that you started in the second stage of the plan should have increased your stamina as well. And the strengthening exercises you started this month should be starting to tone up your body.

If you've not reached your goal, it's time to think about why not. Was the goal unrealistic? Hoping to lose more than 1–2lb a week is probably unrealistic and unhealthy. You may have fallen short of your goal but have still lost weight.

If you have not been sticking to the plan, you may not have lost as much weight as you'd like. Go back and remind yourself of the basics, make those changes, and then you will see a result. It doesn't matter if you haven't achieved it yet, start eating in a healthy way and moving your body and you will lose weight, even if it takes a while longer than 12 weeks.

Progress chart

Date	(__/__/__)	(__/__/__)			(__/__/__)	(__/__/__)
	ORIGINAL	CURRENT			ORIGINAL	CURRENT
Weight			Flexibility scores	1.		
Chest				2.		
Waist				3.		
Hips				4.		
Others				5.		
_____				6.		
_____				7.		
_____				8.		
			Healthy eating score			

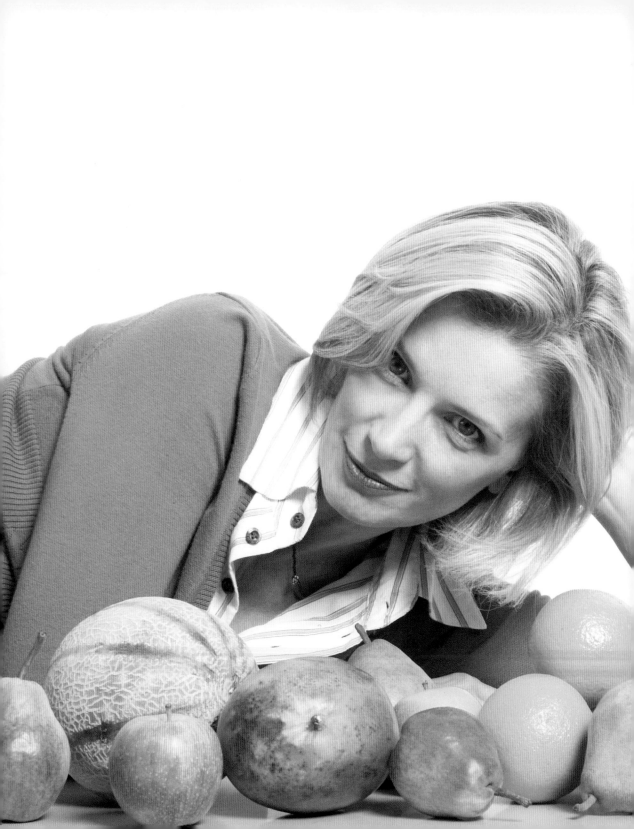

CHAPTER 6

Cook up a treat

We thought you'd like to try some of our favourite recipes. The three of us all have different ways of cooking and eating. You will probably be able to work out who contributed which recipes.

'Coming from a family with origins in Pakistan, I often cook spicy dishes and curries. Although traditionally these recipes may be high in saturated fat and salt, I was taught to cook them by my father, a doctor specializing in heart diseases. He has adapted traditional recipes to make them healthier, but without taking away any of the flavours. My European mother grew up during the war years with rationing, when families had to be very inventive with cooking to stave off the boredom of a very restricted, but healthy, diet. I guess I've fused the two cultures!' **DR SAMINA**

PAM is a working mother, cooking for a family: 'All of the recipes I've contributed here are ones that I cook for myself and my family. Everyone in the family has different tastes but if I keep it as varied as possible I can usually accommodate everyone. I have to bear in mind that my husband needs to keep his cholesterol in check, my teenage son "hates fish" but will indulge me at least once a week, and his sister is famous for pushing the vegetables aside. The recipes are not "health food" meals but really tasty food that happens to be healthy. I include lentils, pulses and grains as well as lean cuts of meat and, of course, the superfoods – fish and vegetables.'

It's different again for **DR BEN**. He eats meat when he's at restaurants, but only cooks vegetarian meals. After a packed day fitting in work and sport, most of the meals Dr Ben cooks are quick and simple – fast food with a difference! 'I usually cook twice as much as I need, so that I can eat the other half the next day, or freeze it to use later. I don't tend to use recipes as such – I experiment, throw it all in together and hope for the best! I can't live without homemade soups. They're so easy and quick to make – and usually good to freeze – and great to use when you can't be bothered to cook. I've got a blender that makes it easy to whiz everything up directly in the pan. I'd encourage you just to give it a go – get cooking with seasonal vegetables and have fun in the kitchen.'

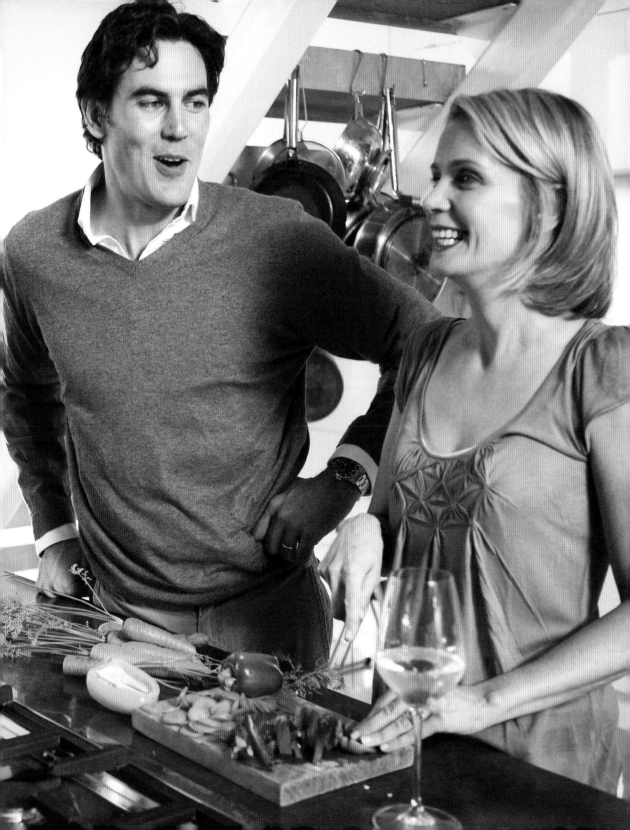

Shakes & smoothies

Berry tasty smoothie

Cool and sweet to slip down easily.

3 large strawberries
100g (3½ oz) frozen strawberries,
   blueberries, raspberries or a
   mixture of frozen berries
115ml (4fl oz) skimmed milk
115ml (4fl oz) natural yoghurt
1 tsp flax seeds
1–2 scoops whey protein

Put all the ingredients in a blender, whiz
and then enjoy!

SERVES 1

Pineapple and banana shake

Another good way to start the day if you really can't face eating breakfast.

½ ripe banana
2 slices of pineapple (fresh is best, but use tinned in fruit juice if more convenient)
60ml (2fl oz) apple juice (or juice from the pineapple tin)
½ tsp flaxseed oil
1 scoop of soya protein
230ml (8fl oz) water

Blend everything together and drink immediately.

SERVES 1

Kiwi, yoghurt and sesame seed shake

A power-packed way to start the day.

1 pear
1 handful of grapes
1 lemon, peel cut off
1 kiwi fruit, halved and contents scooped out
3–4 brazil nuts
1 tbsp sesame seeds
2–4 tbsp natural yoghurt

Using a blender, whiz all the ingredients together until you have a smooth mixture.

You can add 1–2 tbsp wheat germ or oatmeal for some extra magnesium and vitamin E.

SERVES 1

Dips and spreads for snacking

Avocado mash

One of Dr Samina's favourites for breakfast, spread on wholegrain toast.

1 ripe avocado
1 tomato, finely chopped
1 clove of garlic, finely diced
2 slices of white onion, finely diced
Juice of $\frac{1}{2}$ lemon
Black pepper, to taste

Mash the avocado flesh with a fork or blender, and mix with the other ingredients, adding a pinch of black pepper for flavour.

Serve immediately.

SERVES 1

Ben's pesto dip

Good with raw vegetables or served with oatcakes.

2 handfuls of fresh basil
2 tbsp olive oil
1 clove of garlic
Small handful of pine nuts
Black pepper, to taste

Whiz all the ingredients together using a blender.

The dip can be stored for a few days in the fridge in a screw-top jar.

SERVES 2

Samina's tapenade

Tasty spread on oatcakes, rice cakes, crispbreads or wholegrain toast, or serve with a salad.

300g (10½ oz) pitted black olives
200g (7oz) capers
100g (3½ oz) anchovy fillets (use tinned for convenience, but wash the fillets thoroughly first)
A pinch of dried thyme or a sprig of the fresh herb
1 bay leaf
1–2 cloves of garlic, crushed
125g (4½ oz) olive oil, plus a little extra for sprinkling

Place all the ingredients, except the olive oil, in a blender. Whiz everything together then gradually add the olive oil.

Serve immediately, or store for a few days in a bowl covered with a dribble of olive oil.

SERVES 2

Chickpea dip

Another of Dr Samina's toast toppings for breakfast, and makes a tasty snack during the day.

395g (14oz) tin of chickpeas, drained and rinsed
1 clove of garlic, finely diced
Juice of ½ lemon
1 tbsp olive oil
Diced chilli pepper, to taste
Black pepper, to taste

Mash the drained chickpeas and mix in the garlic, lemon juice and olive oil, adding chilli and black pepper to taste.

SERVES 2

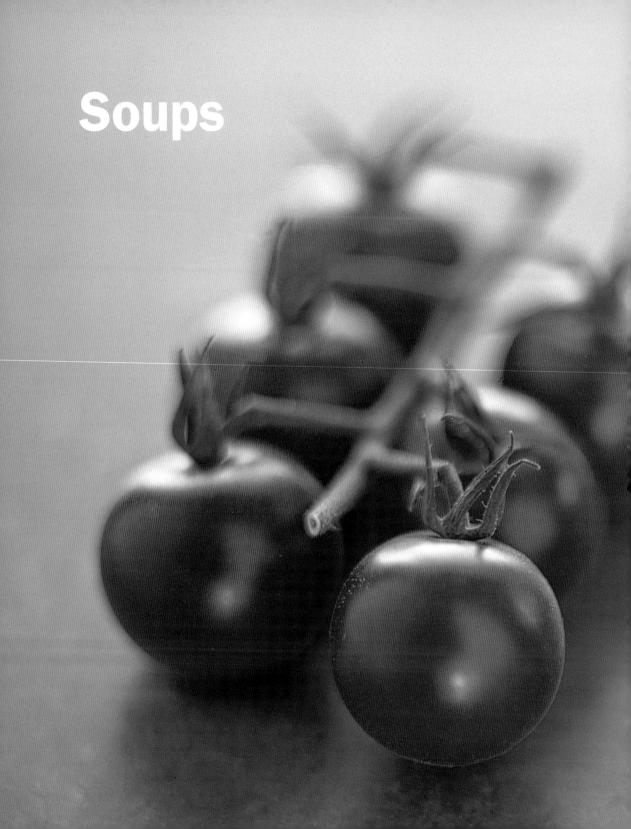

Soups

Roast tomato and basil soup

Easy to make and good to freeze – a soup that can also be used as the base for a pasta sauce.

6 tomatoes (doesn't matter what type, just make sure they're red and ripe)
Pinch of dried mixed Italian herbs
Dash of olive oil
3 cloves of garlic
½ large onion
750ml (26fl oz) vegetable stock (made with hot water and a vegetable stock cube for convenience)
Handful of fresh basil leaves
Pinch of cracked black pepper

Preheat the oven to 170C/325F/Gas Mark 3.

Halve the tomatoes and place on a baking tray, cut side up, and sprinkle with the Italian herbs and a dash of olive oil. Add the garlic and onion to the baking tray, too, leaving their skins on. Roast for about 30 minutes or until the tomatoes start to brown slightly. Remove from the oven and place the tomatoes in a saucepan, including all the juices. Squeeze the garlic and onion out of their skins and into the saucepan. Mix everything together, then pour in the vegetable stock and simmer on a low heat for about 10 minutes.

Whiz the soup in a blender until you have a smooth consistency, adding more stock if needed. Finish by stirring in chopped fresh basil leaves and cracked black pepper.

SERVES 2

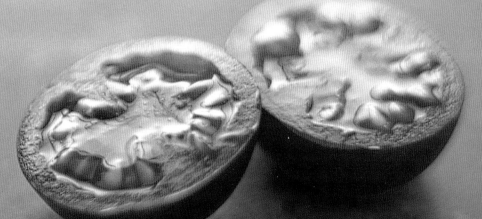

Easy minestrone

A good soup for a tasty and nutritious lunch.

1 onion, sliced
1 clove of garlic, crushed
1 stick of celery, chopped
Olive oil
125g (4½ oz) mixed dried beans, such as borlotti, black-eyed, butter, kidney, haricot or flageolet, soaked in water overnight, or a tin of these beans, rinsed
1 tsp dried Italian herbs
2 tomatoes, chopped
395g tin (14oz) chopped tomatoes
750ml (26fl oz) vegetable stock (made using hot water and a vegetable stock cube for convenience)
Handful of wholemeal spaghetti, broken into bite-size pieces
1 handful of chopped courgettes, carrots and mushrooms
Handful of basil, chopped
Handful of flat-leaf parsley, chopped
Salt and pepper, to taste

Simmer the onion, garlic and celery in a dash of olive oil until transparent. Add the beans, Italian herbs, tomatoes, tinned tomatoes and vegetable stock and simmer for around 30 minutes until the beans are cooked through.

Add the pasta and cook until *al dente*, then add the vegetables – make sure to not overcook them.

Finish off the soup by mixing in the basil and parsley, and seasoning with a pinch of salt and pepper.

SERVES 2

Red lentil, carrot and chilli soup

Colourful and spicy – hot in every way!

$^1/_2$ **onion, diced**
1 clove of garlic, thinly sliced
Olive oil
2 carrots, scrubbed but not peeled,
   tops and bottoms chopped off
125g (4$^1/_2$ oz) dried red lentils
$^1/_4$ **tsp mixed dried cumin**
$^1/_4$ **tsp dried ginger**
$^1/_4$ **tsp dried coriander**
750ml (26fl oz) vegetable stock
   (made with hot water and a
   vegetable stock cube for
   convenience)
$^1/_2$ **red chilli, thinly sliced**
Handful of fresh chopped coriander

Simmer the onion and garlic with a dash of olive oil until soft, then add the carrots, lentils and mixed dried herbs and spices. Mix all together and cover with vegetable stock – you'll need quite a bit of stock as the lentils absorb a lot of fluid. Boil until the carrots are cooked and the lentils look slightly mushy. Add in the sliced chilli, less or more depending on how hot you like the soup.

Whiz all the ingredients together with a hand blender, and garnish with a handful of fresh coriander.

If you make the soup too hot, add a dollop of natural yoghurt when you serve it, to cool it down a little!

SERVES 2

Borlotti bean soup

Very filling, a good meal that packs in
the nutrients but not the calories.

60ml (2fl oz) olive oil
1 celery stick, finely chopped
1 onion, finely chopped
1 carrot, finely chopped
1 leek, finely chopped
395g (14oz) tinned borlotti beans,
    rinsed, or fresh beans, or dried
    beans soaked in water overnight
Handful of parsley stalks, finely
    chopped
1 garlic clove, crushed
2 cherry tomatoes
750ml (26fl oz) vegetable stock
    (made with hot water and a
    vegetable stock cube for
    convenience)
A few celery leaves
Salt and freshly ground black
    pepper, to taste

Heat the olive oil in a large saucepan.
Add the celery, onion, carrot and leek
and cook until softened.

Add the borlotti beans, parsley stalks,
garlic and tomatoes and bring to the
boil. Reduce the heat, cover and
simmer for 30 minutes (or 50 minutes
if the beans are fresh or an hour and
40 minutes if dried).

Add the celery leaves at the end and
season to taste.

SERVES 2

Lentil soup with spinach

A nutritious soup that's filling and satisfying too – a good lunch to have when friends come round.

1 tbsp olive oil
1 small red onion, finely chopped
Small handful of pancetta or
    unsmoked bacon, sliced or diced
1 clove of garlic, crushed
1 carrot, finely chopped
1 celery stick, finely chopped
1 leek
4 cherry tomatoes, chopped
100g (3½oz) brown or green lentils
    (try Puy lentils for a change)
600ml (21 fl oz) stock (made using
    hot water and a vegetable stock
    cube for convenience)
Handful of spinach
Lemon juice
A few mint leaves, to garnish

Heat the olive oil in a large saucepan and cook the onion until softened. Add the bacon or pancetta and garlic and cook on a moderate heat for a couple of minutes, then add the other vegetables and the lentils and stir around for a minute or so. Add the stock and simmer for about 30–35 minutes until the lentils are cooked.

Wash the spinach and put in a shallow pan over a high heat with the lid on so it can steam in the water left on the leaves from the washing. Leave for 2 minutes then take it out of the pan and drain, squeezing the water out as much as possible. Put the spinach in a bowl and pour the soup on top. Season with lemon juice and garnish with mint leaves.

SERVES 2

Fish

Pam's 'healthy' fish and chips

Just as tasty as a takeaway, but much more nutritious and requires very little effort.

2 large baking potatoes
1 tsp olive oil
2 pieces of fish (such as fillet of cod, haddock, plaice or mackerel)
Knob of butter
100g (3½ oz) frozen peas
Tomato ketchup or low-fat mayonnaise, to serve

Peel the potatoes and halve lengthways, then slice again into 'fat chips'. Put the chips on a baking tray and splash over some olive oil, mixing round to cover well.

Cook at 170C/325F/Gas Mark 3 for about 30–45 minutes, shaking the chips around regularly to stop them sticking to the tray.

About 10–15 minutes after putting the chips in the oven, start cooking the fish. Put the fillets in a shallow ovenproof dish with the knob of butter. Cover with foil and cook in the oven with the chips. Cook the peas.

Remove the fish and chips from the oven and serve with the peas and tomato ketchup or a little mayonnaise.

SERVES 2

Tuna, rocket and lemon pasta

A filling meal that is good for all the family.

140g (5oz) pasta such as fettuccine
1 tbsp olive oil
1 small clove of garlic, crushed
200g (7oz) tin of tuna in olive oil, drained
Handful of rocket
Salt and pepper, to taste
Zest and juice of ½ lemon

Heat a large pan of water and bring to the boil. Add the pasta and cook until *al dente*.

At the same time, heat the olive oil and add the garlic, but keep on a low heat so that it just sweats – garlic can easily burn.

Add the tuna and mash into the garlic, then stir in the rocket. Season with salt and pepper and add the lemon zest and juice.

Drain the pasta and add it to the sauce, mixing well.

Serve with green beans.

SERVES 2

Linguine with smoked salmon

This meal is a great source of vitamin B12, folate and the minerals calcium, zinc, selenium and iodine.

300g (10$\frac{1}{2}$ oz) cooked pasta, such as linguine

6 asparagus spears, chopped diagonally or 100g (3$\frac{1}{2}$ oz) baby spinach

$\frac{1}{2}$ red onion, finely sliced

1 clove of garlic, crushed

1 tsp olive oil

4 cherry tomatoes, quartered

125g (4$\frac{1}{2}$ oz) smoked salmon, cut into strips

$\frac{1}{2}$ tbsp fat-free yoghurt or low fat crème fraîche

Pinch of celery salt

Salt and pepper

2 tbsp snipped fresh chives or parsley, to garnish

55g (2oz) Parmesan shavings, to garnish

In a large pan of boiling water, cook the pasta and asparagus. Remove the asparagus when just under *al dente*.

Fry the onion and the garlic gently in the olive oil until soft. Add the tomatoes and cook for a further minute. Toss in the asparagus, smoked salmon strips, pasta, yoghurt or crème fraîche and seasonings. Warm through for a minute or so until hot.

Garnish with the chives or parsley, scatter on the Parmesan shavings and serve immediately.

SERVES 2

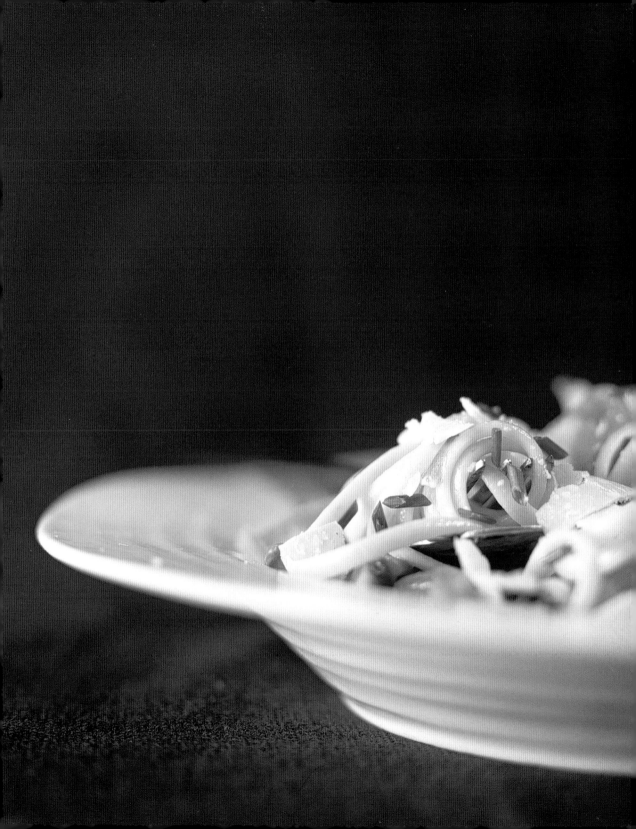

Halibut with lemon

A simple, quick and tasty way to cook white fish. Great served with green beans and potatoes.

Juice of 1 lemon
2 fillets of halibut weighing about 200g (7oz) each
225g (8oz) new potatoes
125g (4½ oz) green beans
40g (1½ oz) butter

Squeeze the juice of the lemon over the fish fillets and leave to soak for 15 minutes while you prepare the vegetables.

Scrub the new potatoes and boil until cooked (15–20 minutes).

Top and tail the green beans, and steam them for a few minutes.

Take the fish fillets out of the juice and dry gently with some kitchen paper. Then gently melt 30g (1oz) of the butter in a large frying pan. Add the fish and cook for about 4 minutes on each side, then transfer to a warmed plate.

Turn up the heat and add the lemon juice used for soaking the fish, and the rest of the butter, and stir while the sauce thickens. Pour over the fish and serve with the new potatoes and steamed green beans.

SERVES 2

Fish curry

A spicy way to serve fish.

300g (10½ oz) cod
½ tsp lovage (or celery seed)
Juice of ½ lemon
Pinch of salt
½ large onion
2 cloves of garlic
Dash of olive oil
75g (2½ oz) Greek yoghurt
½ tsp turmeric
1 tsp red chilli powder
½ tsp garam masala
Handful of coriander leaves,
   to garnish

Marinate the fish in the lemon juice with the lovage and pinch of salt for at least 3 hours, preferably overnight.

Liquidize the onion and garlic in a blender with half a cup of water, then fry over a medium heat with a dash of olive oil, adding another half cup of water and stirring until the onion mixture turns into a golden brown paste.

Stir in the yoghurt, turmeric and chilli powder, then add the fish. Cover the pan with a lid and cook on a low heat. Turn the fish pieces after 10 minutes, using a flat spoon to avoid breaking the flesh. Replace the lid and continue to cook for a further 20 minutes.

Sprinkle the garam masala all over, so that it permeates into the dish, and leave to cook for a further 5 minutes, then garnish with coriander leaves and serve with a side dish of vegetables (such as spinach).

SERVES 2

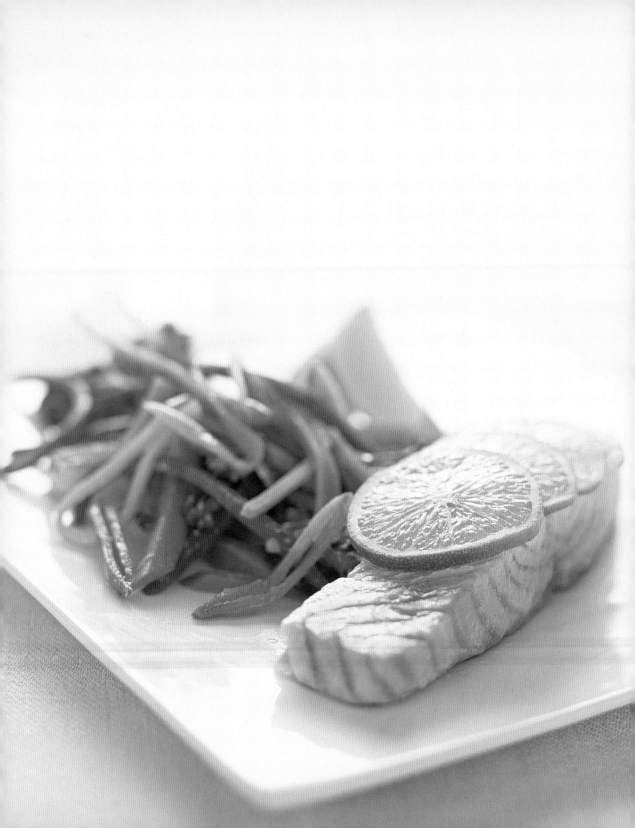

Salmon or tuna parcels with mixed vegetables

A simple dish that keeps all the flavours wrapped in.

2 salmon fillets or tuna steaks,
   each approximately 100–125g
   (3¹⁄₂–4¹⁄₂ oz)
Dash of olive oil
125g (4¹⁄₂ oz) green beans, topped
   and tailed
4 baby carrots, quartered lengthways
¹⁄₄ red onion, finely chopped
8 fresh mushrooms, cleaned and
   sliced
2 tsp fresh flat-leaf parsley
1 tsp melted butter
1 tbsp lemon juice
Salt and pepper

Preheat the oven to 170C/325F/Gas Mark 3.

Cut 4 pieces of aluminium foil or parchment paper into squares big enough to cover each fillet, leaving a border of about 5cm (2 inches), and lightly brush with olive oil. Place the fish in the centre of 2 squares.

Cook the green beans and the carrots in a small amount of water. Drain, then combine in a bowl with the onion, mushrooms and parsley.

Place the vegetable mixture on top of each fish fillet. Drizzle the melted butter and lemon juice over the fish and season lightly. Cover each piece of fish and vegetable mix with another square of foil or parchment, and fold the edges together to form sealed parcels. Bake for 10–15 minutes.

SERVES 2

Fish Pie

A good way to serve fish to children who think they don't like fish!

600g (21oz) peeled potatoes such
   as King Edwards
15g (½ oz) butter
Handful of fresh washed spinach
200g (7oz) white fish such as
   haddock or cod
170ml (6fl oz) skimmed or semi-
   skimmed milk
1 bay leaf
½ onion, finely chopped
Dash of olive oil
½ carrot, finely chopped
1 tbsp plain flour
½ level tsp English mustard
Juice of ½ lemon
1 egg, hardboiled and quartered
Small bunch of parsley, chopped

Preheat the oven to 220C/425C/Gas Mark 7.

Cut the potatoes into quarters, put in a large pan of boiling water and simmer until tender. Drain, and mash with some of the butter. Put to one side.

Steam the spinach in the water clinging to the leaves after washing, and set aside.

Put the fish in a saucepan, cover with the milk and add the bay leaf. Simmer for a few minutes until the flesh turns opaque and the skin can be taken off. Drain off the milk and keep for later. Put the fish into a shallow pie dish.

In a frying pan, slowly fry the onion in the olive oil then add the chopped carrot and cook for a few minutes. Add the flour and stir for a minute or so, then stir in the milk that the fish was cooked in to make a creamy sauce. Add the mustard, lemon juice and parsley.

Put the boiled egg quarters in the pie dish with the fish, add the spinach and pour on the sauce. Add a little more chopped parsley, cover with the mashed potato and bake for about an hour.

SERVES 2

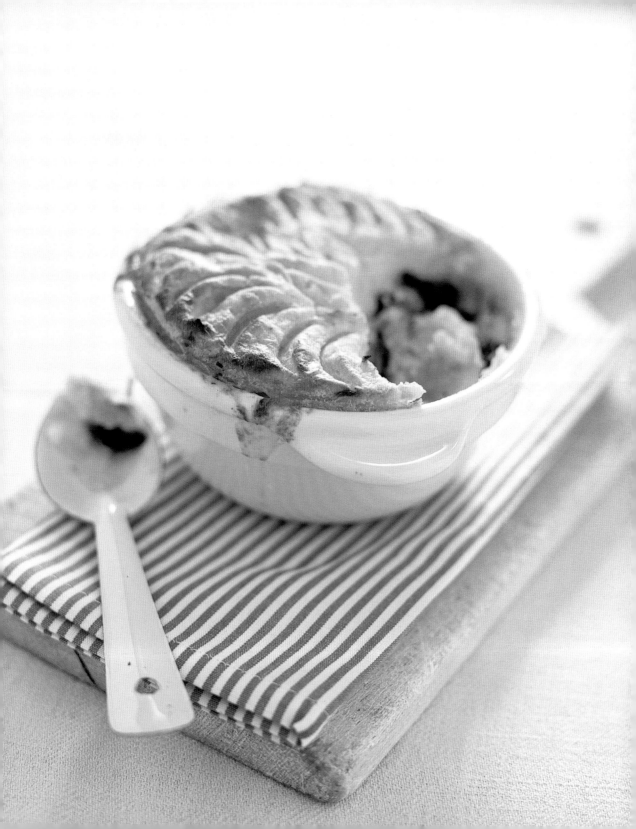

Chicken

Chicken burger

A nutritious version of the fast-food favourite.

200g (7oz) skinless boneless chicken, pounded into 2 flattened pieces
45ml (1½ fl oz) orange juice
1 clove of garlic, crushed
¼ onion, finely chopped
½ tsp dried oregano or thyme
½ tbsp olive oil
Salt and black pepper

Put the chicken in a flat container or plastic food bag and add the orange juice, garlic, onion, herbs, olive oil and seasoning. Seal and refrigerate for about 30 minutes (or if you are thinking about tomorrow, then leave it overnight).

To cook, remove the chicken from the marinade and dry a little using kitchen roll. Grill on each side until the chicken is white all the way through.

Serve with wholegrain burger buns, a green salad and sliced tomatoes.

SERVES 2

Traditional balti chicken

Like a traditional balti dish, this does not contain onions.

2–2.5cm ($^3/_4$–1 inch) root ginger, grated
Olive oil
2 medium tomatoes, sliced
Pinch of salt
$^1/_4$ tsp cumin
1 green chilli pepper, with seeds, finely sliced
1 green chilli pepper, seeds removed, finely sliced
$^1/_4$ tsp turmeric
500g (18oz) chicken, cut into pieces
Handful of coriander leaves, to garnish

Fry the grated ginger in a drop of olive oil for 2–3 minutes.

Add the tomatoes and fry for 4 minutes on a medium heat.

Add the salt, cumin, green chillies and turmeric and fry for 3–4 minutes.

Add the chicken and leave on a low heat for 20 minutes until cooked through.

Garnish with coriander and serve with a vegetable side dish (such as aloo sag), and chapattis or naan bread.

SERVES 2

Paella with chicken and prawns

An easy version of the Spanish classic.

140g (5oz) large raw unpeeled
    prawns, fresh or defrosted if
    previously frozen
500–750ml (18–26fl oz) chicken stock
    (made stock cubes if easier)
3 tbsp olive oil
170g (6oz) chicken, cut into 2cm
    ($^{3}/_{4}$ inch) cubes
1 small onion, finely chopped
2 cloves of garlic, finely chopped
1 large ripe tomato, chopped
70g (2$^{1}/_{2}$ oz) runner or green beans,
    sliced
1 sweet red pepper, seeded and
    cut into strips
140g (5oz) paella rice
Pinch of saffron threads
1 tsp sweet paprika
1 tbsp chopped parsley, to garnish
Lemon wedges, to serve

Peel the prawns. Pour the chicken stock into a saucepan and add the prawn shells and heads. Simmer for 10 minutes.

Heat half the oil in a paella or frying pan and add the chicken. Stir-fry for a couple of minutes on high heat, stirring round to seal all the surfaces. Take out of the pan and put to one side.

In the same pan, heat the rest of the olive oil, add the chopped onion and garlic and cook gently for around 6–7 minutes, then add the tomato, beans and red pepper and continue to cook for a few more minutes. Add the rice to the pan and stir for a minute so the rice gets coated with the oil. Add the hot stock, holding back the prawn shells and heads, and stir. Add the saffron and paprika. Then cover the pan so the rice can cook.

After 10 minutes, add the chicken and prawns evenly over the top of the rice, pushing them under the stock. Cook for a further 5 minutes until the prawns have turned pink. Turn off the heat and leave the paella to sit for 5 minutes before serving with chopped parsley and lemon wedges.

SERVES 2

Chicken with white beans, tomatoes and olives

Chicken with a difference.

2 free-range chicken thighs
8 Kalamata olives, halved
$\frac{1}{2}$ onion, chopped
1 tomato, chopped
$1\frac{1}{2}$ tbsp olive oil
1 tbsp balsamic vinegar
395g (14oz) tin white beans such
   as haricot, drained and rinsed
6 basil leaves, chopped
1 tbsp chopped fresh herbs
1 clove of garlic, crushed

Preheat the oven to 180C/350F/Gas Mark 4.

Place the chicken thighs in a shallow dish and add the olives, onion, tomato, olive oil and half the vinegar. Then cover with foil and bake until the chicken is cooked through (approximately 40–50 minutes).

Put the beans in a pan, add the garlic and cook for a couple of minutes. Add the herbs and the rest of the vinegar and cook for a further 5 minutes or so. Serve with the chicken.

SERVES 2

Karahi chicken

A delicious, colourful dish.

½ **large onion**
3 **cloves of garlic**
Olive oil
500g (18oz) **chicken, cut into pieces**
Pinch of salt
2–2.5cm (¾–1 inch) **root ginger,**
   sliced
¼ **tsp red chilli powder**
¼ **tsp turmeric**
3 **green cardamom pods**
¼ **tsp cumin**
½ **green sweet pepper, seeded and**
   chopped
½ **red sweet pepper, seeded and**
   chopped
1 **large tomato, sliced**
2 **tbsp natural yoghurt**
Handful of coriander leaves, chopped
¼ **tsp black pepper**

Liquidize the onion and garlic in a blender with a cup of water. Heat in a karahi (a thick-based, flat-bottomed pan, similar to a Chinese wok) or a frying pan.

When the onion mixture is beginning to dry out, add a drop of oil and fry over a medium heat until golden brown.

Add the chopped chicken, salt, ginger, spices and black pepper. Cook over a low heat for 20 minutes, until the chicken is cooked.

Add the chopped green and red peppers plus the tomato, with some water if needed, and cook for a further 10–15 minutes.

Stir in the yoghurt and coriander, and serve with naan bread and vegetables.

SERVES 2

Coconut chicken

A very popular dish with the contributors to *The Diet Doctors: Inside and Out.*

200ml (7fl oz) low-fat coconut milk
1 garlic clove, crushed
½ tsp chilli paste
1–2 tbsp chopped fresh coriander
Freshly ground black pepper
1 tsp olive oil
2 skinless chicken breast fillets,
    cut into strips, approximately
    130g (4½oz) each
140g (5oz) brown rice
340ml (12fl oz) vegetable stock
    (made with hot water and a
    vegetable stock cube for
    convenience)
1 small red pepper, deseeded and
    chopped into strips

Place the coconut milk, garlic, chilli paste and coriander with some black pepper into a bowl then add the chicken breast strips to marinate while you cook the rice.

Put the rice in a large frying pan and cover with the stock. Cover with a lid and cook for 25–30 minutes without stirring. Keep covered so that the rice stays warm.

Heat the oil in a frying pan or a wok and pour in the chicken with the marinade, and then cook on a medium heat for about 5 minutes, until the chicken is almost cooked. Add the red pepper strips and cook for another 5 minutes to make sure the chicken is cooked through.

Serve with the rice and steamed broccoli.

SERVES 2

Meat

Meatballs in tomato sauce

FOR THE MEATBALLS

255g (9oz) lean minced beef
¼ large onion, finely chopped
1 tbsp finely chopped parsley
¼ tbsp dried thyme
125g (4½ oz) breadcrumbs
½ dark green apple, peeled and grated
½ tbsp concentrated chicken stock
½ clove of garlic, finely diced
Black pepper

FOR THE SAUCE

¼ large onion
½ large carrot
½ stick of celery
½ clove of garlic
1 tbsp olive oil
1 tbsp apple juice
395g (14oz) tin tomatoes
½ tbsp balsamic vinegar
¼ tsp dried thyme
¼ tsp dried basil
½ tsp dried oregano
½ bay leaf
Salt and pepper

Put the meatball ingredients into a bowl and mix together. Form into 4cm (1½ inch) meatballs, then bake at 200C/400F/ Gas Mark 6 for about half an hour until a little crispy round the outside.

While the meatballs are cooking, make the sauce. Whiz the onion, carrot, celery and garlic together in a food processor, or chop them finely. Heat the oil in a large pan and cook the onion mixture until softened, then add the apple juice, tomatoes and balsamic vinegar. Add the herbs, bay leaf and salt and pepper, to taste, and cook for about 25 minutes on a low heat. Whiz with a hand blender to make a smooth sauce.

Add the cooked meatballs and leave for a few minutes.

Serve with rice.

SERVES 2

Pam's basic mince with hidden vegetables

Cook more to make another, different meal for tomorrow with no extra effort.

1 tbsp olive oil
200g (7oz) lean organic beef, minced
Salt and pepper
½ onion, finely chopped
½ carrot, finely chopped
½ courgette, finely chopped
2 green beans, finely chopped
395g (14oz) tin tomatoes
750ml vegetable stock
Tomato purée
Pinch of nutmeg

Heat a drop of olive oil in a frying pan and add the minced beef. Cook on a high heat for a few minutes until it turns brown. Keep stirring and separating out the meat so that it doesn't bunch together. Season with salt and pepper then transfer to a bowl and set aside. Add some more of the oil to the pan and fry the onion for a few minutes until it softens. Add the vegetables and cook for a few more minutes. Return the meat to the pan, stir then add the tomatoes, tomato purée, nutmeg and the stock. Bring to the boil then cook gently for an hour or so.

Turn the basic mince into shepherd's pie by pouring into an ovenproof dish, covering with a thin layer of mashed potato and baking in a moderate oven for 30 minutes. Make it into a spaghetti sauce by adding a teaspoon of dried Italian herbs. Or add some chopped chilli peppers and a tin of red kidney beans, drained and rinsed, to make a dish with a Mexican flavour.

SERVES 2

Lamb goulash

Quick to prepare then can be left to cook itself.

15g (½ oz) butter
1 onion, sliced
1 dessertspoon paprika
1 clove garlic, crushed
500g (18oz) middle neck of lamb
   (stewing lamb), cut into 2½ cm
   (1 inch) cubes
½ dessertspoon plain flour
90ml (3fl oz) vegetable stock
395g (14oz) tin of tomatoes
1½ tbsp tomato purée
140ml (5fl oz) natural unflavoured
   yoghurt
Chopped fresh flat leaf parsley

Melt the butter and cook the onion, paprika and the garlic, then add the lamb and cook until brown on all sides.

Gradually add the flour and the stock and stir to a smooth sauce.

Add the tomatoes and the purée and simmer gently. You can either let it cook in the pan on the hob, or in a moderate oven for about an hour.

When the meat is cooked, take off the heat, stir in the yoghurt and scatter over chopped parsley.

Serve with red cabbage or carrots, and noodles, rice or potatoes.

SERVES 2

Spicy minced lamb with peas

Pep up the taste buds with a simple lamb curry.

140g (5oz) onions, sliced
1 tsp olive oil
300g (10$\frac{1}{2}$oz) lamb, minced
2 cloves of garlic, sliced
2–2$\frac{1}{2}$cm ($\frac{3}{4}$–1 inch) of root ginger, sliced
Pinch of salt
$\frac{1}{4}$ tsp turmeric
$\frac{1}{4}$ tsp chilli powder
3 green cardamom pods
1 medium tomato, sliced
70g (2$\frac{1}{2}$ oz) frozen peas
Handful of coriander leaves, chopped
Pinch of cumin
$\frac{1}{4}$ tsp garam masala

Fry the onions in a drop of olive oil until golden brown, then add the meat, garlic, ginger, salt, turmeric, chilli powder, cardamom and tomato, adding 2 cups of water. Cook over a low to medium heat for 45 minutes, stirring to prevent sticking and adding more water if it starts to dry up.

Add the peas and cook for a further 5 minutes.

Add the coriander, cumin and garam masala and simmer on a low heat for a few minutes, then serve with vegetables and brown rice.

SERVES 2

Lamb tikka

An easy and healthy version of a takeaway favourite.

300g (10½ oz) lamb meat
(such as leg), cut into cubes
Pinch of salt
2 tomatoes, sliced
2–2½cm (¾–1 inch) of root ginger,
   sliced
1 green chilli pepper with seeds,
   sliced
½ green chilli pepper without seeds,
   sliced
1 tsp olive oil
1 tbsp yoghurt
Handful of chopped coriander leaves

Cook the lamb with the pinch of salt and a cup of water over a medium heat for 30 minutes, adding more water as it dries up.

Add the sliced tomatoes, ginger and chilli peppers and cook over a low to medium heat for a further 15 minutes without adding more water. When the meat is cooked, add the olive oil and fry on a medium heat for a few minutes before garnishing.

Stir in the yoghurt and chopped coriander and leave over a low heat for a few minutes.

Serve with aloo sag, chapattis or naan bread, and a vegetable side dish.

SERVES 2

Healthy burger

Pam's nutritious version of the fast-food favourite.

250g (9oz) extra-lean beef, minced
¼ onion, grated
¼ tbsp Worcester sauce
Black pepper and salt

Mix together all the ingredients and form 2 burgers about 2½cm (1 inch) thick.

Grill on both sides until cooked through, then serve on a wholewheat burger bun with sliced tomato, lettuce and sliced Spanish onion.

SERVES 2

Vegetarian

Easy pizza

Pam's quick and nutritious version –
why not let the children have fun
making their own.

1 ready-made wholemeal pizza base
from health-food shop or supermarket

SERVES 2

For the tomato sauce

$1/2$ medium onion, finely chopped
$1/2$ tsp dried oregano
1 clove of garlic, crushed
200g (7oz) can chopped tomatoes
1 tbsp tomato purée
Freshly ground black pepper

Mushroom and green pepper topping

2 mushrooms, thinly sliced
$1/2$ green pepper, thinly sliced
$1/2$ red onion, thinly sliced
30g (1oz) low-fat mozzarella cheese,
   thinly sliced

Mozzarella with sun-dried tomato topping

55g (2oz) sun-dried tomatoes
30g (1oz) low-fat mozzarella cheese,
   thinly sliced
6 black olives
Small handful of fresh basil leaves

Hot red onion topping

30g (1oz) low-fat mozzarella cheese, thinly sliced
1 red onion, thinly sliced
2 jalapeño peppers, chopped
Pinch of Cajun pepper
1 tsp dried oregano

Preheat the oven to 220C/425F/Gas Mark 7.

Blend all the ingredients for the tomato sauce in a food processor or using a hand blender.

Spread the sauce on the base. Add a topping, then bake for 10 minutes.

Serve half a pizza per person, with a green salad.

Florentina topping

30g (1oz) low-fat mozzarella cheese, thinly sliced
55g (2oz) steamed spinach
Pinch of nutmeg
1 tsp dried oregano
1 egg, broken into the centre of the pizza

Green risotto

Colourful and fresh looking – summer on a plate!

½ tbsp olive oil
½ onion, chopped
½ stick of celery, finely chopped
55g (2oz) runner beans, topped and tailed
Vegetable stock cube
1 clove of garlic, chopped
200g (7oz) risotto rice
40ml (1½ fl oz) white wine
55g (2oz) baby spinach
55g (2oz) petit pois or peas
2 tbsp chopped herbs such as parsley, mint and chives
100g (3½ oz) Parmesan shavings

Heat the olive oil in a frying pan and add the onion and celery. Stir and cover for about 6 minutes.

Cook the runner beans in boiling water for 5 minutes and set aside, but keep the liquid, topping it up to 1 litre (1¾ pints) and adding a vegetable stock cube. Bring to the boil and keep warm.

Add the garlic and rice to the pan with the onion and celery. Stir and then add the white wine. Continue stirring until the wine has been absorbed.

Add the hot stock a ladleful at a time. When nearly all the stock has been used, add the spinach, peas or petit pois, cooked runner beans and herbs. Cover and let it stand for about 5 minutes.

Season with salt and pepper and serve topped with Parmesan shavings.

SERVES 2

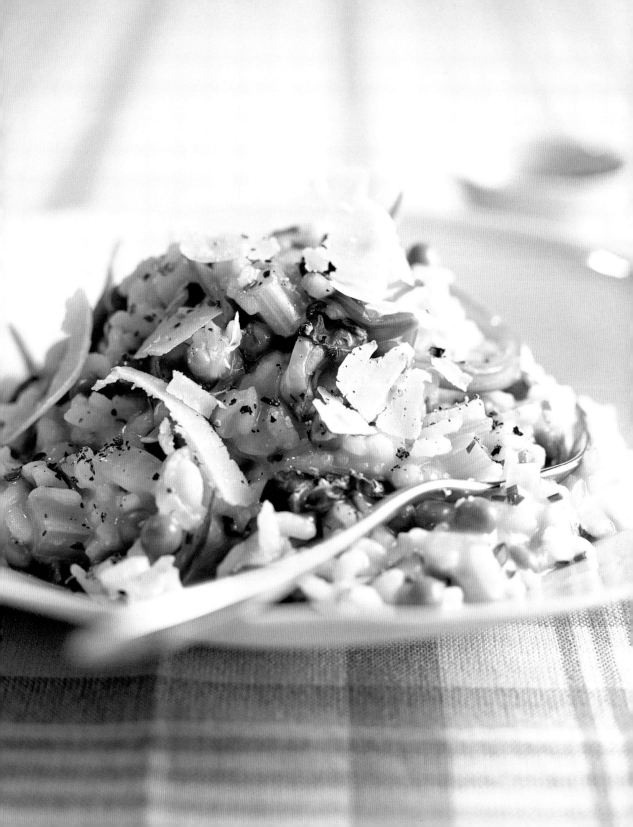

Linguine with sweet potato, feta and rocket

One of Dr Ben's favourite suppers.

1 medium-sized sweet potato
Salt and pepper
Olive oil
1 small red onion
1 tbsp honey
Vegetable stock (made using hot
    water and a vegetable stock cube
    for convenience)
170g (6oz) pasta, such as linguine
30g (1oz) feta cheese
2 handfuls of rocket

Preheat the oven to 170C/325F/Gas Mark 3.

Peel and chop the sweet potato into bite-sized chunks, place on a baking tray and season with salt, pepper and olive oil. Bake the sweet potato for 20–30 minutes until it starts to brown and is soft all the way through.

Thinly slice the red onion and simmer in a pot on a low heat with a dash of olive oil and water until the onion starts to soften. Add honey and stir. The onion will start to caramelize and taste sweet. Add a small amount of vegetable stock to the onion to make it less sticky – you want it to be easily pulled apart to mix through the pasta.

Cook the pasta as per the packet instructions. When the pasta is cooked, drain and then place back in the pot. Stir the sweet potato, red onion, feta and rocket through the pasta.

SERVES 2

Pasta with aubergines and peppers

A healthy alternative to a meat-based pasta sauce.

170g (6oz) linguine pasta
1 tbsp olive oil
1 small chilli pepper
100g (3½ oz) aubergine, cut into
  cubes
1 small onion, chopped
1 red or orange bell pepper,
  deseeded and sliced
2 cloves of garlic, crushed
395g (14oz) tin of chopped
  tomatoes
1 tsp fresh thyme

Heat the oil in a large pan and cook the whole chilli pepper for about 2 minutes. Remove the chilli from the pan, discard the stem and the seeds, and chop the rest of the pepper into small pieces.

Add the aubergine to the pan and cook for a few minutes until browned, then add the onion, bell pepper and garlic, and cook for about 5 minutes. Then add the tomatoes and the chilli pepper. Bring to the boil then reduce the heat to a simmer and then add the fresh thyme. Simmer for about 10–15 minutes until the vegetables are cooked and the sauce thickens.

Meanwhile, cook the pasta as instructed on the packet.

Drain the pasta and mix with the sauce.

SERVES 2

ABC salad

A tasty mix of avocado, artichoke, beans and cashew nuts.

1 medium avocado, peeled, stoned
   and sliced
55g (2oz) radish, cut into thin
   wedges
170g (6oz) tinned or jarred
   artichoke hearts in brine, halved
4 cherry tomatoes, halved
14 raw cashew nuts
55g (2oz) haricot beans
100g (3½ oz) mixed leaves
55g (2oz) black or green olives
1 tbsp olive oil
3 tbsp orange juice

In a bowl, mix together the avocado, radish, artichoke, tomatoes, nuts, beans, leaves and olives.

Combine the olive oil and orange juice in a small jug then pour over the salad.

SERVES 2

Green bean and pimiento salad

Quick and easy to prepare.

500g (18oz) French beans, topped
   and tailed
2 tbsp red wine vinegar
4 tbsp olive oil
200g (7oz) pimiento from a jar,
   finely chopped
1 small red onion, finely chopped
2 medium eggs, hardboiled, shelled
   and roughly chopped

Cook the beans in boiling water, then drain and transfer to a salad dish.

Make the dressing by combining the red wine vinegar and olive oil. Pour over the beans.

Add the other ingredients, finishing with the eggs.

SERVES 2

Seasonal roasted vegetables with yoghurt couscous

A colourful and tasty dish.

2 handfuls of seasonal chopped vegetables, such as red onion, garlic, sweet potato, asparagus, aubergine, red and yellow sweet pepper and courgette
1 tbsp olive oil
170g (6oz) couscous
1 handful of chopped coriander
Juice of ¹⁄₂ lemon
2 tbsp natural yoghurt

Preheat the oven to 170C/325F/Gas Mark 3.

Coat the chopped vegetables in a small amount of olive oil, place on a baking tray and then roast for half an hour or until the vegetables are soft in the middle.

Place the couscous in a bowl and pour over boiling water so that it is just covered. Using a fork, fluff the couscous up, place a tea towel over the bowl and let it sit for 10 minutes.

Stir the coriander, lemon juice and yoghurt into the couscous.

Place the couscous on a plate and layer the roasted vegetables on top.

SERVES 2

Arabic feast

Another quick meal from Dr Ben, good when entertaining friends.

'Search out a food store that specializes in Arabic or Middle Eastern food, or check out the deli section of your supermarket, and stock up on freshly made chickpea dip, smoked aubergine dip, spinach leaves, fresh coriander, pitta bread, freshly made falafels, halloumi, couscous salad, tomatoes, parsley salad, olives and anything else that looks fresh and healthy. Warm up the falafels, dry-fry the halloumi in a pan until brown and soft in the middle and then place on a platter with the other ingredients so you can graze on it, either making a salad or a sandwich with the pitta bread.'

Baked sweet potato with cottage cheese

A vitamin-packed alternative to a baked potato.

1 medium sweet potato
Drop of olive oil
2 tbsp cottage cheese or low-fat goats' cheese
2 spring onions, sliced

Preheat the oven to 180C/350F/Gas Mark 4.

Scrub the sweet potato and dry with paper towel. Place on a baking sheet and rub with olive oil. Bake for 30–40 minutes or until soft and tender.

Cut open and add the cheese and spring onions.

Serve with cherry tomatoes and green salad.

SERVES 1

Lentil curry in a hurry

Lives up to its name.

200g (7oz) tin of brown lentils, washed and drained
½ bay leaf
½ tsp cumin seeds, lightly crushed
½ tsp coriander seeds, lightly crushed
½ onion, sliced
1 tbsp olive oil
½ clove of garlic, crushed
1cm (½ inch) fresh root ginger, chopped finely
½ red bell pepper, deseeded and cut into fine strips
½ courgette, cut into 2cm (¾ inch) cubes
¼ tsp turmeric
Handful of fresh coriander, chopped
½ tsp garam masala
4 cherry tomatoes, quartered
Salt and pepper, if needed

Put the lentils, bay leaf, cumin and coriander seeds in a pan with 285ml (½ pint) water and bring to the boil. Turn down to a simmer and cook for 15 minutes. Drain and put aside.

Fry the onion in half the oil for about 5 minutes until golden brown, then set aside.

Put the rest of the olive oil in the pan and then add the garlic, ginger, pepper and courgette and cook for about 4 minutes.

Add the cooked lentils, turmeric, fresh coriander, garam masala and cherry tomatoes and heat through, seasoning with salt and pepper if necessary.

Serve with the caramelized onion on top, with naan bread or rice.

SERVES 2

Desserts

Grilled mango

One of Dr Ben's favourite desserts when entertaining friends.

1 mango
½ tbsp brown sugar
Crème fraîche to serve

Cut the mango in half lengthways, removing the stone.

Score crisscross lines across the flesh with a knife.

Sprinkle with brown sugar and place flesh side up under a hot grill, until the sugar begins to caramelize.

Remove from the grill and serve with a blob of crème fraîche.

SERVES 2

Fresh fruit salad

Popular with Dr Samina, Pam and Dr Ben, as part of breakfast, a handy snack or a dessert.

Chop up and combine any fresh fruit you have available. Dr Ben likes a combination of raspberries, blueberries, strawberries, blackberries, orange, melon, banana and passion fruit.

Cinnamon baked apple with cranberries

A good warm winter pud.

1 large baking apple
115ml (4fl oz) unsweetened apple
   juice
30g (1oz) dried cranberries
¼ tsp powdered cinnamon

Preheat the oven to 200C/400F/Gas Mark 6.

Cut the apple in half and remove the core.

Pour 60ml (2fl oz) of the apple juice into an ovenproof dish and place the apple cut side down in the juice. Bake for 20 minutes or so until the apple is cooked.

Meanwhile, simmer the rest of the apple juice for 5 minutes. Add the cranberries and the cinnamon, reduce the heat and simmer for a further 10 minutes.

Serve the apple halves in individual serving dishes cut side up, with the cranberry mix spooned over.

SERVES 2

Strawberries dipped in chocolate

A chocolate hit without overdoing the calories!

A small punnet of strawberries
55g (2oz) good quality dark
   chocolate, minimum 70 per cent
   cocoa solids

Wash and hull the strawberries.

Melt the chocolate in a small bowl over a saucepan of hot water.

Dip the strawberries in the chocolate, to cover half the fruit and leave half exposed. Place on greaseproof paper to harden.

SERVES 2

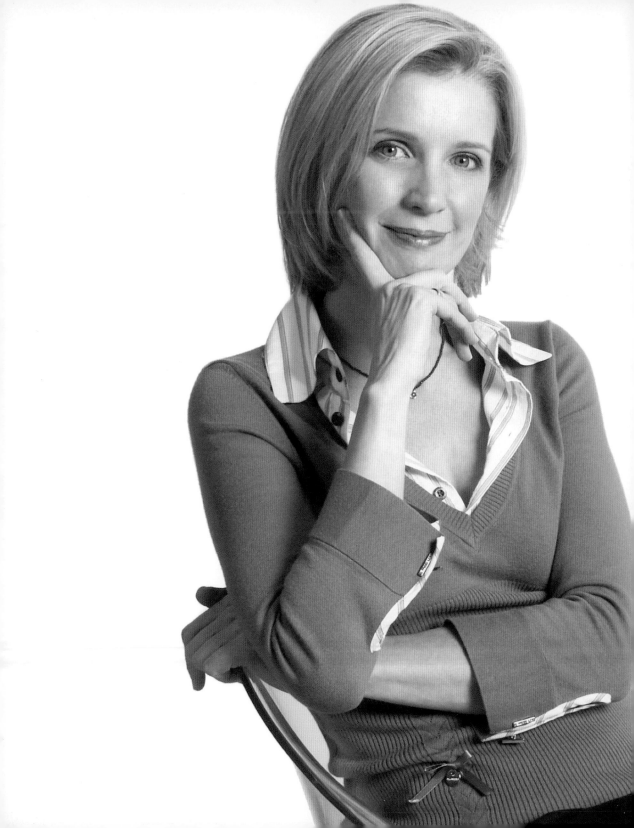

CHAPTER 7

What next?

So what's next? You've reached the end of the 12-week diet plan, which means you've finished, right? Sadly, it doesn't work that way. If you had more than a stone to lose, then you'll need to carry on with the plan if you are going to reach your ultimate goal. Even if you've reached your target weight, you will need to carry on if you are going to stay slim for life.

Hopefully, you've enjoyed the 12-week plan. It should now be second nature to fit in your 10,000 steps a day along with your range of movement exercises for maximum flexibility. Regular cardiovascular and strengthening exercise should be part of your life now too.

Foodwise, your body should be used to eating three nutritious meals, with healthy snacks, to banish hunger. You should now be eating at least five portions of fruit and vegetables each day, including wholegrains in your diet, and getting at least two portions of fish a week. Eating like this, you're doing the best you can for your inside, with benefits showing through on the outside. Why throw it away?

So how are you going to maintain the weight loss you've already achieved? It's a good idea to think about why you want to stay with the new slimmer you. Remind yourself of all the changes that you've made that have allowed the weight to drop off. Carry on with your new eating and exercising patterns and you will continue to reap the benefits. Your weight will continue to drop and your health to improve. But go back to your old habits and the weight will creep back on. It's also a good idea to think about what might stop you sticking to healthy eating and regular exercising. Then you can plan how you are going to avoid these danger zones.

You might find it helpful to get rid of all the clothes that are now too big for you. If you start putting on weight, you won't want to go out and buy bigger clothes again. Another idea is to take the photograph of the new slimmer you and stick it somewhere prominent (like the door of the fridge) and next to the original photo you took at the start of the plan where you look larger. This will remind you why you want to stay slim for life.

'When I'm helping patients maintain their weight loss, I always tell them to set a limit a few pounds above their current weight and decide never to cross that line. If their weight hits the limit, then they know it's time to take further action! That's when they need to think about portion sizes – it's easy for portions to creep up and the next thing you know, the pounds are coming back on. It's also easy for the odd nibble or extra snack or second glass of wine to slip back in. If you reach the limit, then it's time to cut back on portions and cut out the extras until you are safely back at the weight you want to be. If you genuinely don't know why the weight increase has happened, then keep a food diary again to help you spot what's happening. But one thing's certain – if you don't weigh yourself regularly, and by that I mean once a week, you won't spot that things are slipping!' **PAM**

So our final message to you is to keep going. Make being healthy on the inside a way of life, so that you can continue to look good on the outside. That way you will also feel great and stay slim for life.

Appendix

If you are concerned about any of the symptoms listed below, you should visit your GP.

PROBLEMS WITH HEALTH	MAKE THESE CHANGES TO THE 12-WEEK DIET PLAN

SKIN

If you often have ulcers, sores or fungal infections

In Pam's experience, sores and ulcers may indicate a shortage of vitamins A and C, so increase the amount of orange fruit and vegetables you eat (such as carrots and tomatoes), citrus fruits (such as orange and grapefruit) and green leafy vegetables (such as cabbage, spinach and watercress). They can also indicate an immune system problem so a blood test to check your blood count is worthwhile should any persist more than 3 weeks or be recurrent. Mouth ulcers can also reflect inflammatory bowel conditions so do see your GP. If you suffer regularly from any type of skin problem, including fungal infections, spots or boils, then it might be worth asking your doctor to check your blood sugar levels to rule out diabetes.

If your skin is often greasy and spotty

Spotty and greasy skin may be helped by cutting down on excessive fats, such as those found in crisps, chips and pork pies, and increasing vegetables. Greasy or spotty skin, particularly if associated with irregular periods, excessive hair growth and weight gain, is likely to be a sign of polycystic ovarian syndrome (PCOS). It is important to have this diagnosed by your GP. In some cases symptoms can be eased by cutting out chocolate and refined sugar from your diet.

If your skin bruises easily

Frequent nosebleeds and bruising easily may be the first sign that the 3 certain vitamins, especially vitamin K and C, which is found in abundance in green leafy vegetables such as spinach and citrus fruits. Abnormal bruising may also be caused by problems with the liver or even the blood itself and any concerns should be addressed by your GP.

PROBLEMS WITH HEALTH	MAKE THESE CHANGES TO THE 12-WEEK DIET PLAN
If your skin often itches, or is dry and flaky	This can be an indication of an allergic skin condition, eczema or psoriasis. This might be helped by foods rich in vitamins B2, B6 and biotin, such as green leafy vegetables, wholegrain cereals, eggs and dairy produce. You might also be short of essential omega unsaturated oils, so increase the amount of seeds, nuts and oily fish (such as sardines, mackerel, tuna, whitebait) that you eat.

HAIR

If you've got excessive hair loss	Hair loss all over the head may be due to iron shortage or thyroid problems, while patchy hair loss might need an antifungal treatment or be a result of hormone imbalance, so check with your doctor. You could try eating more liver, red meat and green leafy vegetables to boost iron. Increasing B vitamins by eating more wholegrain cereals and eggs may help, and increase zinc intake by eating more shellfish. There may also be insufficient protein in your diet – more likely in vegetarians and vegans. Stress and pregnancy can also trigger hair loss.
If your hair has changed in amount or texture	Dry hair may be a sign of a shortage of vitamins A or B6, so eat more orange fruits and vegetables (like carrots and pumpkins), green leafy vegetables and eggs. Dry hair can also be a symptom of an under-active thyroid.

FINGER AND TOE NAILS

If your nails have changed in appearance, shape or texture	Thickened nails can be a sign of a fungal infection, which can be cleared up with medication from your doctor. Ridges on the nails can indicate a shortage of iron so make sure your diet includes lean red meat and green leafy vegetables such as spinach. If not due to knocks, spots on the nails could mean a shortage of zinc so eat more shellfish and seeds.
If your nails are brittle or often peel or break	If the problem's not due to having your hands in water too long, it could be due to a shortage of zinc or iron, so beef up your intake of lean red meat, liver, eggs, green leafy vegetables, shellfish and seeds. Severe calcium deficiency can result in brittle nails, so give your dairy intake a boost.

PROBLEMS WITH HEALTH	MAKE THESE CHANGES TO THE 12-WEEK DIET PLAN

EYES

If your eyes feel dry or itchy	Dry eyes might be helped by increasing your intake of vitamin B2, found in green leafy vegetables and dairy produce, while itchy eyes might indicate allergy so eat foods that help to reduce inflammation, like oily fish, fresh pineapple, ginger, nuts, garlic and berries, but steer clear of spicy food and caffeine.
If you experience difficulty seeing when it is dark or have night blindness	This might indicate a shortage of vitamin A, so increase the amount of carrots and other orange fruits and vegetables that you eat.
If there are any raised yellow bumpy spots around your eyes or a white ring round the coloured part of your eye	These are both signs of raised cholesterol levels. Have your fasting cholesterol checked, and, if raised, cut back on the amount of processed food and meat you eat (to reduce saturated fats), and have more oily fish and nuts (to boost unsaturated fats) and soluble fibre (found in oats, beans and pulses).

MOUTH/THROAT

If your gums bleed when you clean your teeth	This is often a sign of gum disease, or gingivitis, although it might also be a symptom of scurvy. You may have a shortage of vitamin C, so increase the amount of green leafy vegetables and fruit that you eat.
If your breath smells unpleasant	This can be a sign of a poor diet, excess stomach acidity and reflux. This should improve as you follow the diet plan. Eating natural yoghurt can be particularly helpful.

PROBLEMS WITH HEALTH	MAKE THESE CHANGES TO THE 12-WEEK DIET PLAN
If there's a scummy look to your tongue, or it's red and cracked	White patches on the tongue can indicate yeast overgrowth, so eat natural yoghurt and probiotics, and cut out refined sugar. A purplish tongue can indicate shortage of vitamin B2 (so eat more green leafy vegetables and dairy produce) or biotin (so eat more liver, nuts and brown rice) and too much alcohol (so cut it out for a while). A red shiny smooth tongue can indicate a shortage of vitamins B3, B12 and folic acid (so choose more wholegrains, green leafy vegetables, dairy produce, eggs, avocados, apricots, pumpkin and Marmite). If your tongue is pale, it can indicate you are short of iron so beef up the red meat and liver in your diet.

POSTURE, STANDING HOW YOU USUALLY STAND

If the back of your head is not in line with your heels, your backside or belly stick out, your shoulders jut forwards, your hips are at different levels or one leg looks longer than the other	If your posture is poor, check out pages 66–67. Pay particular attention to the exercises given for Weeks 1–4. They will help you stretch out your body and improve your posture. If your posture has not been corrected after four weeks, you could visit a chiropractor to ensure good alignment within your body before you progress to the next stages of the exercise plan.

HEART AND CIRCULATION

If you have high blood pressure	It is important that you lose weight and reduce salt intake to below 6mg/day.
If you have high cholesterol levels	Restrict saturated fat intake by cutting back on animal products (butter, meat) and eat more oily fish and nuts. Eat more foods with soluble fibre (such as oats, beans, pulses).
If you've ever had heart or circulation problems	Again reduce your salt intake and animal fats. Magnesium is essential for a healthy heart, so make sure that you include plenty of magnesium-rich foods in your diet, such as whole grains, nuts, brown rice, tofu and kelp.

PROBLEMS WITH HEALTH	MAKE THESE CHANGES TO THE 12-WEEK DIET PLAN

DIGESTIVE SYSTEM

If you suffer from heartburn or indigestion

Don't eat late at night, avoid spicy food and caffeine, keep alcohol and smoking to a minimum. Make sure you eat three small meals each day with two snacks between, so that you don't feel too full or too empty. Try to address any stress issues as well.

If you often have diarrhoea or constipation

You may have irritable bowel syndrome so ensure you have small but regular meals, eaten in a calm environment when you are not stressed, and do not skip the snacks. Some people respond well to increasing the fibre in their diet, while it makes symptoms worse in other people – so experiment! Having a probiotic often helps. You may also be suffering from a food sensitivity or intolerance. Common culprits are lactose and gluten.

If there's ever blood in your stool

If you have piles or a cut near the anus caused by straining, eating more fibre will be helpful, though you should also always discuss the problem with your doctor.

If you have diabetes

You are at higher risk of developing heart and circulation problems, so reduce salt intake and the amount of animal products you eat, and increase the amount of oily fish, nuts and leafy green vegetables instead. Keep to a low-sugar diet.

MUSCLES AND BONES

If you have muscle cramping or pain

You might be short of the essential minerals, calcium and potassium, so increase the amount of fruit, vegetables and dairy produce (such as milk, yoghurt and cheese) that you eat. If symptoms persist, see your GP.

If you have muscle weakness

You might want to bring forward the third stage of the exercise plan, aimed at improving muscle strength, but make sure you don't push yourself too hard. You might also benefit from eating foods rich in iron such as lean meat, spinach, prunes and liver.

PROBLEMS WITH HEALTH	MAKE THESE CHANGES TO THE 12-WEEK DIET PLAN
If you have osteoporosis or bone fractures	Bone health is improved by a diet rich in calcium (so that means lots of milk and other dairy produce, or drinks enriched with calcium) and vitamin D (made in the skin by sunlight, or eaten in foods such as oily fish and eggs). Try goats' or sheep's milk or soya milk if you don't like cows' milk. Eat foods rich in magnesium, manganese and zinc (so lots of nuts, seeds, wholegrain cereals and shellfish). Building up muscle strength helps balance which can reduce falls, so you might want to make an early start on the strengthening exercises (given in Week 9). Your GP can advise you if you need to take any medication.
If you have arthritis or joint problems	Make sure that you eat enough foods containing vitamin E (found in nuts, seeds, eggs and brown rice) and vitamin C from green leafy vegetables. Cutting back on drinks containing caffeine and spicy food may help.

OTHERS

If you are often tired or fatigued	Doing more exercise can actually give you more energy, so you might want to start the second and third parts of the exercise programme straight away. Tiredness can often be a symptom of iron deficiency anaemia, an underactive thyroid gland or depression. After ruling them out with your GP make sure that your diet is not lacking foods rich in the B vitamins and magnesium. Tiredness can also be caused by too little or poor quality sleep. Avoid eating large meals and drinking caffeine or alcohol late at night.
If you suffer from headaches	These may be caused by too much caffeine, so gradually reduce the amount of tea, coffee and cola drinks you are having. If you suddenly stop all these drinks, your headaches may get worse for a few days before they start improving. Cutting down on cheese, chocolate, citrus fruits, Chinese food, alcoholic drinks (particularly red wine and beer), artificial sweeteners and ice cream may help. Seeing a chiropractor to address tension in the neck can also reduce headaches in some people. See your GP to diagnose any medical cause.

PROBLEMS WITH HEALTH	MAKE THESE CHANGES TO THE 12-WEEK DIET PLAN
If you have weakness or tingling in your fingers or elsewhere	This can be a sign of too little vitamin B1 in your diet, so make sure you choose meals that include lots of wholegrain cereals and eggs. A chiropractor can help if the symptoms are due to a trapped nerve. You should also consult your GP.
If you have low libido	This may improve as you start to lose weight and feel better about your body, though it's also true that lots of thin people have low libido. Exercise can help. You may also benefit from eating foods rich in vitamin B3 such as wholegrain cereals, green leafy vegetables and eggs. Depression, the menopause and taking the Pill can affect your libido, too. Consult your GP if you are worried.
If you often feel depressed or irritable, and find it hard to concentrate	Feeling better about yourself as you start to lose weight and get more active can really help your mood. Following the 12-week diet plan should also help if vitamin and mineral shortage are part of the problem. You might also benefit from taking a RDA dose multivitamin supplement to get you back into balance quickly. If you suspect your levels of iron and vitamin B12 may be low, you may want to ask your doctor to check these levels, or try eating more red meat, eggs and dairy produce. Anti-depressants can sometimes help so consult your GP.
If your weight has changed markedly in recent years	Linked with other signs, such as tiredness or changes in hair growth, weight increase may indicate hormonal problems that your doctor can check (see above). You need to make sure that your diet provides less energy than you need, so that you can lose weight, and eat foods rich in vitamins necessary for hormone regulation, such as liver, shellfish, eggs and wholegrain cereals.

Acknowledgements

Dr Samina, Pam and Dr Ben

We wish to express our appreciation and thanks to each of the following:

Dr Diane Storey, who gathered together the various strands of expertise and wove them into a coherent narrative; her diligence, patience and skills were greatly appreciated.

The Tiger Aspect production team, who were uniformly professional and supportive: Jo McGrath, Isabelle Gunner, Rebecca Mulraine, Jake Cardew, Clair Satwell, Melissa Mayne, Nicola Tremain, and all of the *Diet Doctors: Inside and Out* team – you were each and every one brilliant, and we had lots of fun. We would also like to thank all of the contributors to the series, who trusted us and were enthusiastic in their endeavours to achieve their goals.

Susanna Abbott, our excellent editor at HarperCollins, whose enthusiasm, support and guidance were constant throughout the entire project. And thanks to Jacqui Caulton for her impeccable design work, Sally Potter and the team at HarperNonFiction. We are also really appreciative of the very fine creative work of Mark Read for his lovely photographs, and make-up artist Paul Xavier and stylist Alex Reid for the glamour!

With thanks to our patients and colleagues from our respective clinics: HSGP, King Chiropractic and The Green Room, and to our friends for inspiration, love and support. Many thanks to Dr Mansur Ahmad, Dr Rhodri Jones, and Dr Nick Miller for their medical expertise.

Last and first and always, a huge thanks to our respective family members: Rodney, Georgia, Richard, Eve and Barney – notwithstanding a huge welcome to the beautiful baby Amelia who was with us all the way.

Tiger Aspect Productions

Tiger Aspect Productions would like to thank all those who have made this not only such a fantastic book, but a fantastic project to work on: the *Diet Doctors: Inside and Out* presenters, Ben, Samina and Pam; Diane Storey, for her invaluable work; all those who have been involved at HarperCollins, and particularly Sally Potter and Susanna Abbott; Jo McGrath, Isabelle Gunner, Rebecca Mulraine, Rhodri Jones and everyone on the *Diet Doctors: Inside and Out* production team; Gordon Wise at Curtis Brown; and Jamie Munro, Jenny Spearing and Elaine Foster at Tiger Aspect.

HarperCollins Publishers

HarperCollins Publishers would like to thank Rigby and Peller; The Park Club, West London; Mark Read, photographer extraordinaire; Rachel Jukes, Stylist, Fergal Connolly, Home Economist; Jo McKenna for additional hair and make-up; and model Fiona Brattle and her family for looking after us so well on location. Special thanks also to everybody at Tiger Aspect Productions, particularly Jo McGrath and Rhodri Jones; Gordon Wise; and of course Pam, Samina, Ben and Diane. It's been great fun.

Index